MEDICAL PARASITOLOGY

A Self-Instructional Text

MEDICAL PARASITOLOGY

A SELF-INSTRUCTIONAL TEXT

EDITION 4

RUTH LEVENTHAL, PhD, MBA, MT (ASCP)
Professor of Biology
The Milton S. Hershey Medical Center
The Pennsylvania State University
Hershey, Pennsylvania

RUSSELL F. CHEADLE, MS, MT (ASCP)
Program Director, MLT
Associate Professor of Medical Technology
University of Rio Grande
Rio Grande, Ohio

ILLUSTRATIONS BY ELLIOT HOFFMAN

F. A. DAVIS COMPANY · Philadelphia

F. A. Davis Company
1915 Arch Street
Philadelphia, PA 19103

Printed in the United States of America

Last digit indicates print number: 10 9 8 7 6 5 4 3 2 1

Acquisitions Editor: Jean-François Vilain
Developmental Editor: Ralph Zickgraf
Production Editor: Roberta Massey
Cover Designer: Steven Ross Morrone

As new scientific information becomes available through basic and clinical research, recommended treatments and drug therapies undergo changes. The authors and publisher have done everything possible to make this book accurate, up to date, and in accord with accepted standards at the time of publication. The authors, editors, and publisher are not responsible for errors or omissions or for consequences from application of the book, and make no warranty, expressed or implied, in regard to the contents of the book. Any practice described in this book should be applied by the reader in accordance with professional standards of care used in regard to the unique circumstances that may apply in each situation. The reader is advised always to check product information (package inserts) for changes and new information regarding dose and contraindications before administering any drug. Caution is especially urged when using new or infrequently ordered drugs.

Library of Congress Cataloging in Publication Data

Leventhal, Ruth.
    Medical parasitology : a self-instructional text / Ruth Leventhal,
Russell F. Cheadle. — Ed. 4.
        p.   cm.
    Includes bibliographical references and index.
    ISBN 0-8036-0041-0 (alk. paper)
    1. Medical parasitology—Programmed instruction.   I. Cheadle,
Russell F.   II. Title.
    [DNLM: 1. Parasitology—programmed instruction.   QX 18.2 L657m
1995]
QR251.L38   1996
616.9'6'0077—dc20
DNLM/DLC
for Library of Congress   95-4649

Preface to the Fourth Edition

Since the publication of the first edition of *Medical Parasitology,* various social and medical phenomena have increased the incidence of parasitic disease among North Americans. Increased world travel by United States citizens and the recent influx of immigrants to this country from underdeveloped regions have brought once-seldom-encountered parasites to our shores. Changes in sexual behavior have altered the epidemiology of infections such as giardiasis and amebiasis. Finally, the advent of acquired immune deficiency syndrome (AIDS) has unleashed previously rare opportunistic parasites such as *Pneumocystis carinii.* Such conditions lend a new urgency to the diagnosis and treatment of parasitic diseases by physicians and the detection of these diseases by technologists. We believe, now more than ever, that all health professionals need a fundamental understanding of the diagnosis, treatment, and prevention of parasitic disease. We have approached our revision with this belief in mind.

Medical Parasitology is designed to provide the reader with a concise, systematic introduction to the biology and epidemiology of human parasitic disease. The text is supported throughout by an array of carefully coordinated graphics. Many of the changes incorporated in this revision are based on responses from surveys of the users of the previous editions. The presentation of the symptomatology, pathology, and treatment of each parasitic disease has been expanded. New unicellular parasites have been added, most notably those associated with AIDS. Information concerning arthropods' roles as ectoparasites has been enhanced, and coverage of serologic testing has been strengthened.

Enhancements to the graphic elements of the text have not been neglected. Line drawings of newly added parasites have been included and previous drawings modified as necessary. All laboratory procedures have been updated and expanded to conform to current quality control standards. Finally, pedagogical improvements include expanded end-of-chapter post-tests and updated bibliographies.

Ruth Leventhal
Russell F. Cheadle

Preface to the First Edition

There are many available textbooks about parasitology. Some of these treat the biology of parasites in great depth, while others are more graphic in nature. The laboratorian or clinican needs both kinds. This book was designed to provide a concise description of the biology and epidemiology of human parasites, coupled with an extensive series of color photographs and line drawings to facilitate visual recognition of parasites found in clinical specimens. Furthermore, several modes of graphic presentation have been incorporated in order to aid the various approaches to learning and mastering the requisites.

This book resulted from our recognition of the need for a self-instructional text in parasitology. Present formal course instruction in medical parasitology is often limited and generally is not designed to allow for different learning styles. Russell Cheadle conceptualized and wrote the original draft of this self-instructional text, while the research and writing thereafter became a truly collaborative effort. The product is, we believe, a useful learning tool for students in biology, medical technology, medicine, and public health, as well as an effective pictorial reference book for the clinical laboratory.

We wish to thank Catherine Cheadle, Mary Stevens, and Valerie Fortune for their kind assistance. Russell Cheadle would also like to thank Dr. Herbert W. Cox, his graduate advisor, for his encouragement.

Ruth Leventhal
Russell F. Cheadle

Contents

Color Plates

The series of color photographs included with this text was selected to show clearly the morphologic and diagnostic characteristics of parasites of medical importance. A brief review of major disease symptoms, the life cycle of the parasite, and other pertinent information are included in the discussion of each photograph. Try to describe each diagnostic stage aloud, recalling the key features of each organism as labeled on the life cycle diagram, to assure yourself that you recall these features.

The Nematoda are a diverse group of roundworms, existing as both free-living and parasitic forms. They vary greatly in size from a few millimeters to over a meter in length. These organisms have separate sexes, and body development is complex. Of the nematode species parasitic for humans, about half live as adults in the intestine, and the other half are tissue parasites in their definitive host. The pathogenicity in intestinal infections may be due to biting and blood sucking (e.g., hookworms, *Trichuris*), to allergic reactions caused by substances secreted from adult worms or larvae, or to migration through the body tissues. Tissue nematodes, the Filarioidea, live in various tissue locations in the host. These organisms require an arthropod intermediate host in their life cycle. The produced pathology varies with the location of the parasites in humans but may involve the occlusion of the lymphatics (*Wuchereria*, *Brugia*), localized subcutaneous swellings or nodules (*Onchocerca*, *Dracunculus*), or blindness (*Onchocerca*).

1,2. *Enterobius vermicularis* (pinworm). 1. Adult male (20 ×) and 2. female (10 ×). These mature in the anterior portion of the colon. The adult yellowish-white female worms are 8 to 13 mm and the male worms 2 to 5 mm in size. Each has a bulbar esophagus as well as finlike projections, called cephalic alae, about the anterior end. Male and female worms are further differentiated in that the male has a sharp curvature of the tail and small posterior copulatory spicule, whereas the female has a long, straight, sharply pointed tail. When the uterus is gravid with eggs, the female migrates from the colon (usually during sleeping hours of the host) to the perianal area, where she deposits her eggs and dies. The adult may also migrate to the appendix, where it can be found histologically. Pinworm disease is essentially an allergic reaction to the release of eggs and other secreted materials from the gravid female that causes severe rectal itching.

3. A higher-power view of the anterior end of the adult, clearly showing the alae.

4. Note the caudal curve and copulatory spicules of the male *Enterobius vermicularis*.

5. *Enterobius vermicularis* eggs (400 ×). Eggs may be recovered from the perianal folds by applying the sticky side of cellophane tape to the skin surfaces and then taping the cellophane, sticky side down, onto a microscope slide for examination. Eggs are rarely recovered in feces. The eggs are elongated (55 μm × 25 μm) and tend to be flattened on one side. The thick shell is transparent and colorless, and the folded larva may be seen within. Pinworm eggs are infective for the host within a few hours of being released. Scratching of the perianal region allows transfer of the eggs by hand to the mouth of the host. The eggs hatch soon after they are swallowed and develop to mature worms within 2 weeks. Bedding, night clothing, and even house dust may be sources of egg infection for others through ingestion or inhalation of airborne eggs. This is a very common parasitic infection in this country and spreads easily, so that those living with an infected individual are likely to become infected.

6. *Enterobius vermicularis* egg (900 ×). This view shows an egg under oil immersion; the developed larva can be clearly seen coiled inside the flattened shell.

7. *Enterobius vermicularis* egg (100 ×). A low-power view of the egg as seen on a cellophane tape preparation. Because of the transparency of the eggs, screening of the slides must be carefully performed, using low illumination.

8. *Trichuris trichiura* (whipworm) (4 ×). Adult female, measuring 35 to 50 mm. The anterior ends of both male and female worms are slender and threadlike, but the posterior one-third of the worm is wider. The posterior end of the female appears club-shaped and straight; the male has a 360-degree coiled posterior with two copulatory spicules. The adults in the intestine attach firmly by embedding a spearlike projection at their anterior end into the mucosa of the cecum and proximal colon. Distribution of this parasite is cosmopolitan, especially in moist, warm areas. This is the most commonly reported parasitic infection in this country. Light infections are usually asymptomatic, but heavy infections may cause enteritis and diarrhea with rectal prolapse.

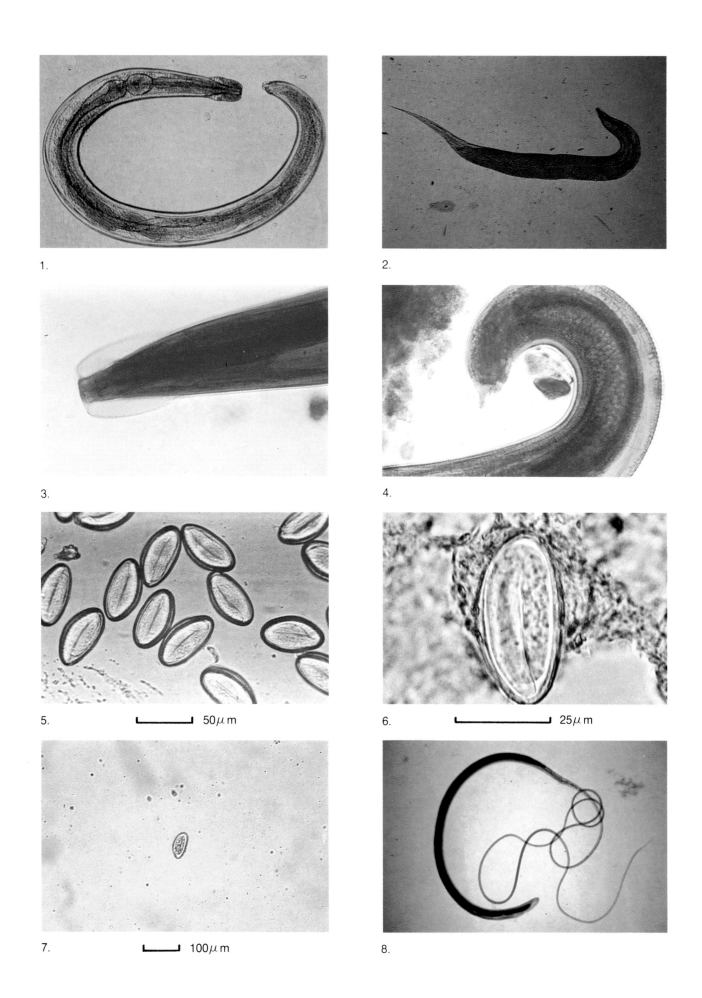

1.

2.

3.

4.

5. ⊢——————⊣ 50μm

6. ⊢——————⊣ 25μm

7. ⊢——⊣ 100μm

8.

9. *Trichuris trichiura* egg (500 ×). Diagnosis: recovery of eggs in feces. Concentration technique needed to detect a light infection. The *Trichuris* egg is characteristically barrel-shaped and measures 20 μm × 50 μm. Note the undeveloped embryo; the clear, inner shell; the heavy, golden outer shell; and the transparent hyaline plugs at the ends of the egg. Eggs passed in feces must remain in a favorable soil environment for at least 10 days until larval development is complete; at this time the egg is infective. Ingestion of the egg from infected soil or contaminated food is followed by hatching in the intestines. The larva molts and develops in the intestines to become an adult. About 90 days are needed for a complete cycle from egg ingestion to egg output by the adults.

10. *Trichuris trichiura* egg. This view shows an egg at a magnification of 100 ×. (Note: Dog whipworm is an occasional zoonosis; egg is much larger [35 μm × 80 μm] and broader.)

11. *Ascaris lumbricoides*. Both male and female adults are shown. They are large, pinkish-white, and conically tapered at the anterior end. A female measures 22 to 35 cm in length by 3 to 6 mm in diameter and has a pinkish-white and straight tail. A male measures 10 to 31 cm by 2 to 4 mm and has a sharply curved tail with two copulatory spicules. The adults live in the small intestine and can survive for over a year. Females lay up to 250,000 eggs per day, which are passed in the feces and can be readily recovered by routine fecal examination. Passage of adult worms from the rectum is often the first indication of infection. Light infections are asymptomatic. Heavy infections may cause pneumonia early in the infection and, later, diarrhea, vomiting, or bowel obstruction. Complications such as perforation of the intestinal wall or appendix with resultant peritonitis or obstruction of airways by vomited worms may cause death. Known as the large intestinal roundworm.

12. An obstructed bowel from a heavily infected patient. Distribution of this parasite is worldwide, although it is more frequently found in tropical areas.

13. *Ascaris lumbricoides* egg (400 ×). Diagnosis: recognition of eggs (or adults) in feces. The fertilized egg measures 40 μm × 55 μm and contains an undeveloped embryo. This egg appears round, but *Ascaris* eggs are slightly oval. The outer coat is albuminous and mamillated; occasionally, eggs without coats may be found (decorticated). The thick, inner coat is of clear chitin. These characteristics are diagnostic. On reaching warm, moist soil, larvae develop within the egg shells in 2 to 3 weeks, and eggs are then infective for humans. Infection occurs by ingestion of these infective eggs in contaminated food or drink. It is not uncommon for *Ascaris* and *Trichuris* to coexist in the same person because of the same method of infection and the requirements for egg development in the soil. Eggs hatch in the intestine, and the *Ascaris* larvae rapidly penetrate the mucosal wall. They reach the liver and then the lungs via the blood circulation. Larvae emerge from the circulation into the lungs in about 9 days, migrate up the bronchi to the esophagus, and are swallowed. They mature in the intestine in about 2 months. In an immune individual, most larvae are destroyed in the liver.

14. *Ascaris lumbricoides* egg. This view shows an egg at a magnification of 100 ×. Ascarids of dogs and cats (*Toxocara* spp.) can undergo partial development and produce pathology in humans. After ingestion of an egg from soil, the *Toxocara* eggs hatch, and the larvae penetrate the intestinal wall and enter the blood circulation but are unable to complete the migratory route. They lodge in tissues and cause inflammatory reactions leading to occlusions of capillaries of vital organs (e.g., eye, liver, brain, lungs). Symptoms vary, depending on the location of the parasite and the host's reaction to it. The disease is called visceral larval migrans. It is seen most commonly in children because they are more likely to ingest eggs from infected soil, such as at a playground where dogs are walked. High eosinophilia is a very common sign. Diagnosis is made serologically or by observing larvae in histopathologic sections. Species identification is difficult but can be done.

15. *Ascaris lumbricoides* egg (400 ×). An unfertilized egg. Note the elongated shape and the heavy, albuminous, mamillated coat. This type of egg is not uncommonly seen.

16. Adult male hookworm (10 ×). Adult hookworms are small, grayish-white nematodes. The anterior end is tapered and curved and has an open buccal capsule. The posterior end of the male terminates in a fan-shaped copulatory bursa and spicules. The raylike pattern of the chitinous supportive structure in the bursa is different for each species. Females (12 mm × 0.5 mm) are larger than males (9 mm × 0.4 mm). The female has a straight and pointed tail and produces 5000 to 10,000 eggs per day. She may live up to 14 years.

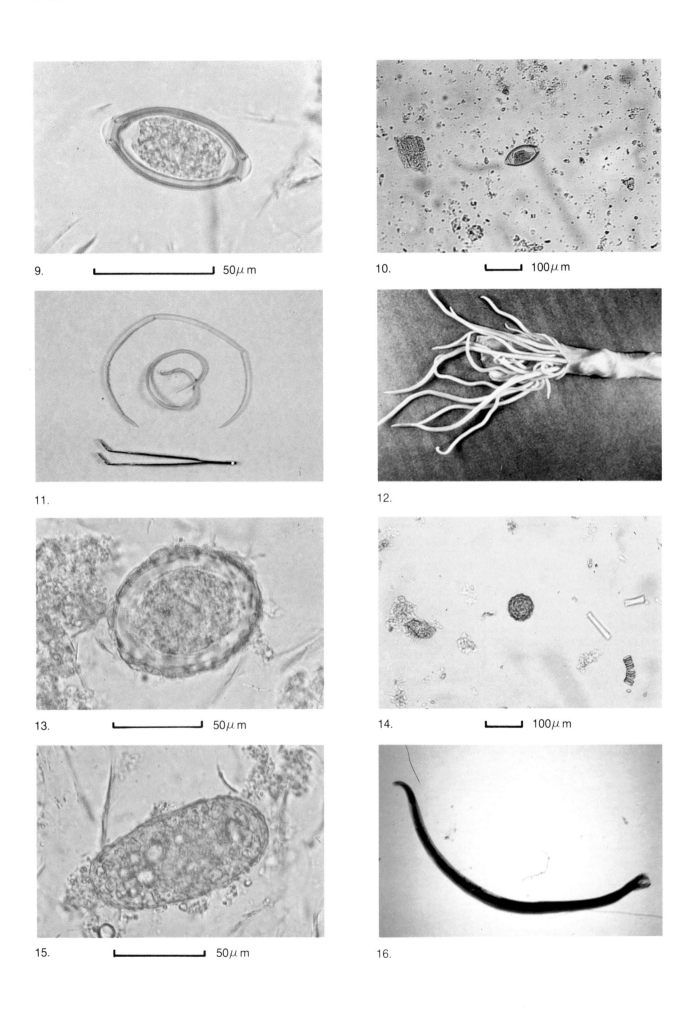

9. |———————| 50μm

10. |———| 100μm

11.

12.

13. |———————| 50μm

14. |———| 100μm

15. |———————| 50μm

16.

17. *Necator americanus* (New World hookworm). The anterior end of an adult worm. Species identification is helped by examining the buccal capsule. Note the pair of semilunar cutting plates in the upper side of the buccal cavity. There is also a second, smaller set of plates on the lower side.

18. *Ancylostoma duodenale* (Old World hookworm). The anterior end of an adult worm. Note the two pairs of teeth in the buccal cavity. The mouthparts of hookworms allow for firm attachment to the mucosa of the small intestine and for ingestion of blood. *N. americanus* is found throughout Africa and the southeastern United States; *A. duodenale* is found in southern Europe, northern Africa, the Far East, and the Mediterranean countries. Both are found in parts of Asia, Central and South America, and the South Pacific. Symptoms of the disease depend on the extent of the infection and the nutritional status of the patient and can appear clinically as a hypochromic microcytic anemia because of the bloodsucking activity of worms. Only a heavy infection causes the disease state.

19. Hookworm egg (500 ×). Note the definite but thin shell and the clear area around the embryo. Diagnosis of the presence of hookworms can be made upon recognition of the egg in feces, but adults must be examined for species identification because the eggs and larvae of these worms look alike. Eggs usually contain an immature embryo in the 4- to 8-cell stage of division if feces are promptly examined. Six cells are visible in this embryo. Eggs measure about 30 μm × 50 μm.

20. Hookworm eggs (500 ×). This view shows more mature eggs containing developing rhabditiform larvae. Eggs are shed in feces, and the embryo rapidly develops to a larva in 1 to 2 days. Eggs hatch to liberate rhabditiform larvae, which then further mature in the soil to become infective filariform larvae.

21. Hookworm rhabditiform larva, showing the anterior end of the first-stage larva (500 ×). Although these larvae are not normally seen in fresh fecal preparations, larvae may develop and hatch if feces are not promptly examined. This view has been included so that differential characteristics between hookworm larvae and *Strongyloides stercoralis* rhabditiform larvae may be studied. Note that the buccal cavity of a first-stage hookworm larva is slightly longer than the width of the head, appearing as two parallel lines extending back from the anterior edge of the larva. It has a longer buccal cavity than that of *S. stercoralis*; this is the primary characteristic differentiating the two (see Plate 25). In addition, the genital primordium is not obvious in hookworm larvae but is visible in *Strongyloides* larvae. The hookworm larva measures 250 μm × 17 μm.

22. Hookworm filariform larva (100 ×). Infection occurs when infective stage (filariform) larvae penetrate skin, especially between the toes. The larvae are carried throughout the body via lymphatic and blood circulation. Most larvae emerge from the circulation in the lungs, migrate up the bronchi to the esophagus, and are swallowed. They complete maturation in the intestine in about 2 weeks. Nonfeeding infective hookworm larvae in soil are ensheathed and have pointed tails. A short esophagus extending about one-quarter of the way down from the anterior end is another differentiating characteristic.

23. Infective filariform larvae of dog and cat hookworms, especially *Ancylostoma braziliense*, can invade human skin, producing an allergic dermatitis called creeping eruption or cutaneous larval migrans. Inasmuch as the human is an unnatural host for the animal hookworms, further larval development does not occur. An itching, red papule is produced at the site of larval entry with development of a serpentine tunnel between the epithelial layers produced as the larva migrates. The larva moves several millimeters per day and may survive several weeks or months. This disease is widely distributed and is common in sandy areas on the Atlantic coast from New Jersey to the Florida Keys, along the Gulf of Mexico, and in many parts of Texas. It is also found in the midwestern United States.

24. *Strongyloides stercoralis* (threadworm) (400 ×). This view is of a rhabditiform larva (225 μm × 15 μm) seen in feces. Concentration techniques are helpful because numbers are low. The esophageal bulb is evident at the junction of the esophagus and intestine, which is about one-fourth of the parasite's length back from the anterior end. This is one diagnostic feature that may be used to differentiate hookworm and *Strongyloides* rhabditiform larvae, because this structure is not as prominent in hookworm larvae. Adult parthenogenic female worms (2.2 mm × 50 μm) live in the submucosa of the upper small intestine. Eggs pass through the mucosa, and the rhabditiform larvae hatch in the lumen of the intestine to be shed in feces. The larvae may develop in soil to become infective filariform larvae and penetrate the skin as do hookworm larvae. They may, however, also molt and become infective before they pass in feces and penetrate the mucosa of the colon to cause autoinfection, especially in debilitated or immunocompromised persons. In either case, they travel via the blood-lung route as do hookworm larvae, returning to the intestine to develop into adults. The life cycle of this parasite may also include a free-living cycle in the soil. In this case, rhabditiform larvae molt and develop in 2 to 3 days to become free-living mature adults. The sexually mature free-living male and female mate and produce eggs that develop into filariform larvae, which are infective to humans via skin penetration.

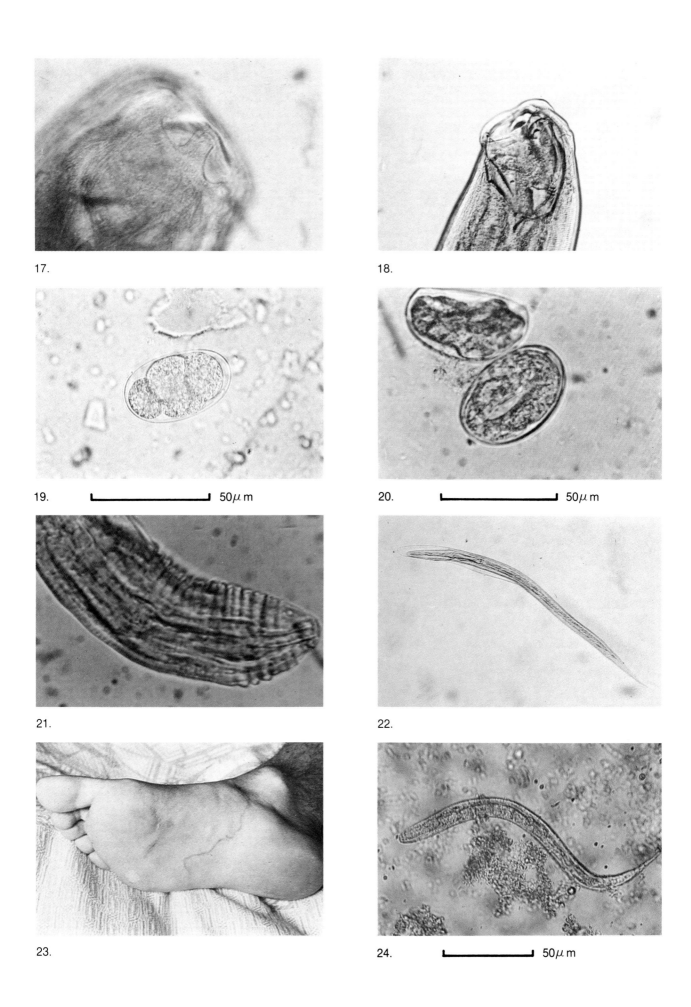

17.

18.

19. |⊢——————⊣ 50μm

20. |⊢——————⊣ 50μm

21.

22.

23.

24. |⊢——————⊣ 50μm

25. *Strongyloides stercoralis* (500 ×). This view shows the short buccal cavity of the rhabditiform larva. The length is one-third to one-half the width of the head of the larva (compare with Plate 21). Diagnosis is based on the recovery of characteristic rhabditiform larvae from feces. The filariform (infective stage) larva of *Strongyloides* recovered from soil or cultured in the laboratory has a notched tail, whereas the filariform larvae of hookworms have pointed tails. This parasite is found worldwide, especially in warm climates. As with hookworm disease, there is a dermatitis at the site of repeated larval entry, and respiratory symptoms may result from the larvae as they migrate through the lungs. Abdominal symptoms vary with the extent of the infection, from mild epigastric pain to vomiting, diarrhea, and weakness with weight loss. Moderate eosinophilia is common. Untreated, the disease may last for many years because of autoinfection from larvae that develop in the colon and may cause death in the immunosuppressed patient.

26. *Trichinella spiralis* (trichina worm). Encysted larva in muscle tissue (400 ×). Adult worms develop (in about 1 week) in the submucosal tissues of the small intestine. They are very small: the male measures 1.5 mm, and the female measures 3.5 mm. Larvae (1 mm) produced by the female pass into the mesenteric venules or lymphatics and are carried throughout the body. Within about 2 weeks they emerge from the blood to enter striated muscle cells or other tissue, although they survive only if they enter striated muscle cells (for instance, in the tongue or diaphragm). The 1-mm larvae become encysted in the muscle and calcify over time but remain alive for years. Many hundreds of larvae may be produced over the female's life span of 2 to 3 weeks. Infection occurs when undercooked pork or bear meat containing encysted larvae is ingested; the larvae develop into adults in the intestines in a few days. The disease state, trichinosis, is found worldwide among meat-eating populations (with the highest prevalence in Europe and North America) and presents a variety of symptoms, including gastric distress, fever, edema (especially of the face), and acute inflammation of muscle tissue. Daily study of blood smears showing increasing eosinophilia is a useful diagnostic aid. A history of eating undercooked meat, skin testing, and positive serologic tests are strongly suggestive of infection but are not conclusive. Definitive diagnosis depends upon demonstration of the encysted larvae in a muscle biopsy from the patient. Attempts at recovery of adult parasites from feces are usually futile. Light infections have vague symptoms, which may be missed.

27. *Trichinella spiralis.* A higher-power view of a stained section. Note the tissue inflammation around encysted larvae in the muscle "nurse cells."

28. *Wuchereria bancrofti* (Bancroft's filaria) microfilaria (400 ×). A thick, peripheral blood smear, stained with Giemsa stain, showing the sheathed embryo, which measures 250 μm in length. The ends of the sheath appear almost colorless and are noncellular, often staining poorly with Giemsa. The presence of a sheath and the pattern of cell nuclei, which can be seen in the posterior end of the microfilaria (upper center photograph), are diagnostic. In this species, a single column of cell nuclei extends only to near the tip of the tail, which has no nuclei. Microfilariae are most prevalent in the peripheral blood at night (nocturnal periodicity); therefore, they are best detected in blood specimens obtained between 9 PM and 3 AM. Blood concentration is helpful. Adult nematodes live in the lymphatics. Prolonged infections cause obstruction of lymph flow, resulting in elephantiasis of the lower extremities, genitalia, or breasts. Other symptoms include fever and eosinophilia caused by allergic reactions to the parasite. *Culex, Aedes, Mansonia,* and *Anopheles* mosquitoes serve as intermediate hosts of *W. bancrofti* and are found in tropical areas worldwide. Diagnosis: recovery of characteristic microfilariae in blood.

29. *Brugia malayi* (Malayan filaria) sheathed microfilaria (400 ×). The sheath stains pink with Giemsa. Note that the nuclei occur in groups to the end of the tail, with two nuclei in the tip (middle right of photograph). These features are diagnostic. The disease produced is essentially identical to *W. bancrofti* but is found primarily in Southeast Asia, India, and China. These microfilariae also exhibit nocturnal periodicity in the blood, and the mosquito vectors are species of *Mansonia, Aedes,* and *Anopheles.* Diagnosis: recovery of characteristic microfilariae in blood at night.

30. *Loa loa* (African eyeworm) microfilaria (400 ×). In this thick blood smear, the sheathed microfilaria can be seen, measuring 250 μm in length. Note that cell nuclei occur in groups through most of the body but are seen in a single line to the tip of the posterior end of the tail (upper right of photograph). This feature is diagnostic. In humans, adults migrate throughout the subcutaneous tissues, causing transient swellings called Calabar swellings. Adults may be seen migrating through the conjunctiva of the eye. Microfilariae are most prevalent in the blood during the day (diurnal periodicity), and the vector is the mango fly (*Chrysops*). The disease is chronic and relatively benign, although allergic reactions may occur, causing edema, itching, and eosinophilia. This parasite is found in West and Central Africa. Diagnosis: recovery of characteristic microfilariae in blood. The sheath does not stain with Giemsa.

31. Children with distinct fibrous nodules on their bodies, which contain adult worms and microfilariae of *Onchocerca volvulus.* The female discharges microfilariae that migrate through the skin but do not enter the blood. The disease is chronic and nonfatal. Allergic reactions to microfilariae cause local symptoms. If microfilariae reach the eye, blindness may occur. This parasite is a major cause of blindness (river blindness) in Africa. Diagnosis is made by excising a nodule with recovery of adult worms or by detecting microfilariae in a tissue scraping of the nodule or a skin snip. When present in the eye, microfilariae may be observed with an ophthalmic microscope. The vector is the blackfly, *Simulium,* which breeds in running water, and the disease is found in Central America, parts of northern South America, and west-central Africa.

32. *Onchocerca volvulus* microfilaria (100 ×) present in a tissue scraping of a skin nodule. The microfilariae are unsheathed and the pointed, often flexed tail contains no cell nuclei. Differentiate from *Mansonella streptocerca* microfilariae, which are also found in skin snips, by the tails, which, in *M. streptocerca,* are bent into button-hook shapes and have nuclei extending into the tips.

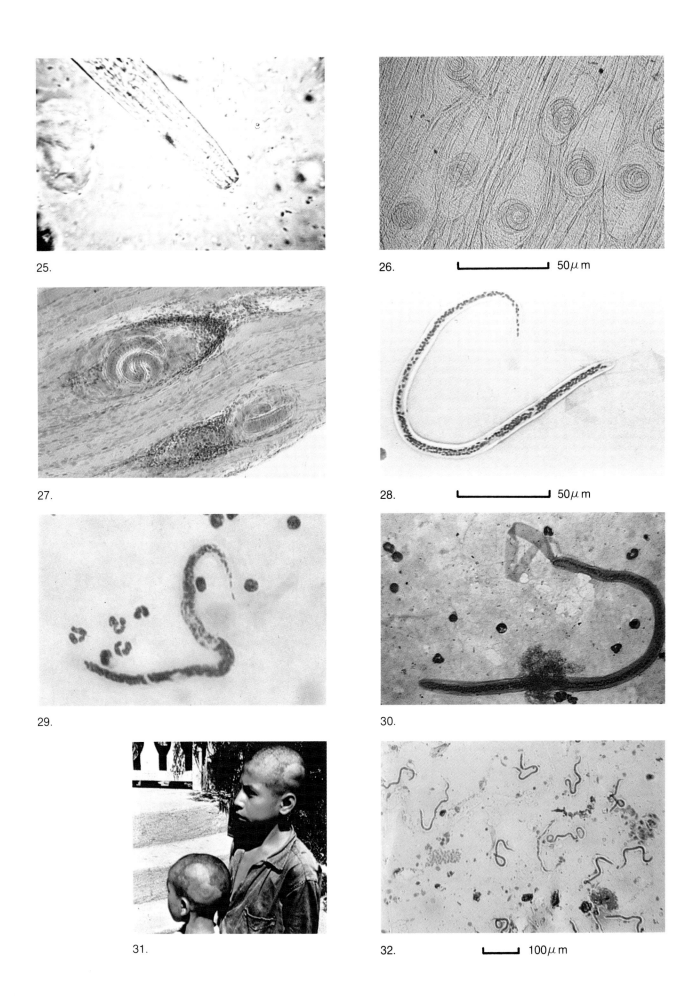

25.

26.   ⊢————⊣ 50 μm

27.

28.   ⊢————⊣ 50 μm

29.

30.

31.

32.   ⊢——⊣ 100 μm

33. *Dracunculus medinensis* (Guinea worm). This view shows part of a female worm protruding from an ulcer and wrapped around a match stick. The female is 70 to 120 cm × 2 mm in length. These worms release larvae into water. Infection occurs when a human drinks water containing crustaceans of the genus *Cyclops* (the intermediate host) infected with a larva of *D. medinensis*. Larvae liberated from the copepods in the human small intestine migrate through the viscera to the subcutaneous tissues and become adults. In the subcutaneous tissues, the female induces an ulcer and releases larvae into water. Larvae released into fresh water penetrate the *Cyclops* intermediate host. The major clinical manifestation of this disease includes allergic symptoms, that is, fever, diarrhea, nausea, eosinophilia, and local symptoms caused by ulcer formation. This parasite is found in the Middle East, Central Africa, the West Indies, and the Guianas. Species that parasitize animals have been found in North America. Diagnosis: detection of the adult in local lesions.

The Cestoda are a subclass of endoparasitic Platyhelminthes (flatworms); the cestodes are commonly known as the tapeworms. The adults live in the intestinal tract of vertebrates, whereas larval forms inhabit tissues of vertebrates or invertebrates. The head (scolex) is modified by suckers and sometimes hooks for attachment to the intestinal wall, and the segments (proglottids), containing both male and female sex organs, bud from the posterior end of the scolex to form the body of the tapeworm (the strobila). The length of tapeworms varies from 2 to 3 mm up to 10 meters. Infection in humans produces primarily intestinal symptoms. Transmission to humans occurs (depending on the species) when insufficiently cooked food containing larvae is eaten or when eggs are ingested.

34. *Hymenolepis nana* (dwarf tapeworm) egg (400 ×). Diagnosis: recovery of characteristic clear, spherical, 30 to 47 μm eggs in feces. Note the threadlike filaments that radiate from two polar thickenings into the area between the embryo and outer shell. Three pairs of hooklets may be seen on the embryo inside the inner shell. Infection is by ingestion of the egg, which hatches in the duodenum. The embryo penetrates the mucosa, where it matures to a cysticercoid larva in the intestinal wall. The larva emerges in a few days and develops to an adult worm. No separate intermediate host is required.

35. *Hymenolepis nana* egg (100 ×). A low-power view of another egg. The rat tapeworm (*H. diminuta*) may also infect humans; the egg is much larger (70–85 μm) and has no polar filaments.

36. *Hymenolepis nana* mature proglottids (100 ×). The proglottid contains a bilobed ovary and three round testes. The testes are visible, but the ovary is not easily seen in this view. Segments are tiny and usually disintegrate in the intestine before passage in the feces. The whole worm measures 2.5 to 4 cm and is the smallest tapeworm to parasitize humans. Multiple infections are common, because eggs can hatch in the intestinal tract and cause an immediate autoinfection as the larvae enter the mucosa. The body of the worm (the strobila) contains about 200 proglottids. Each of these flattened segments contains complete male and female reproductive organs. All nutrient is absorbed from the intestine of the host through the tegument of the tapeworm.

37. *Hymenolepis nana* scolex (100 ×). The small scolex bears four suckers and a retractable rostellar crown with one row of 20 to 30 hooklets. These structures provide for firm attachment to the intestinal mucosa. Light infections may be asymptomatic, but heavy infections produce diarrhea, vomiting, weight loss, and anal irritation. This parasite is found in India and South America and is common in children in the southeastern United States. Autoinfection may occur if eggs hatch inside the host, but usually reinfection is caused by hand-to-mouth transfer of eggs after scratching the irritated anal region.

38. *Taenia* species egg. *Taenia solium* (pork tapeworm) or *T. saginata* (beef tapeworm) egg (400 ×). *Taenia* eggs (30 to 45 μm) are diagnostic for the genus only. Notice the thick, yellow-brown outer shell with its radial striations. The hexacanth embryo inside the eggshell bears six chitin hooklets. The six hooklets are not visible in this view. Eggs of *T. solium* are infective for both pigs and humans. If eggs are accidentally ingested by humans, they hatch, just as they do in pigs, in the small intestine. Larval forms (*Cysticercus cellulosae*) develop in the subcutaneous tissues, striated muscles, and other tissues of the body. Symptoms vary with the location of the cyst. Eggs of *T. saginata* are not at all infective for humans. The source of human infection with the adult pork or beef tapeworm is ingestion of insufficiently cooked pork or beef containing encysted *Cysticercus* larvae. After being digested free, the scolex in the *Cysticercus* everts and attaches to the small intestine, and the larva grows to become an adult in 6 to 10 weeks.

39. *Taenia* spp. eggs (100 ×). This view shows four eggs at low power. Pollen grains may resemble eggs under low power.

40. *Taenia solium* (pork or "armed" tapeworm) scolex (100 ×). Four suckers and a rostellum bearing 20 to 30 large hooks are set in two rows at the anterior end of the scolex. *T. saginata* can be differentiated from *T. solium* because the *T. saginata* scolex does not have hooks, only four suckers, and is therefore said to be "unarmed."

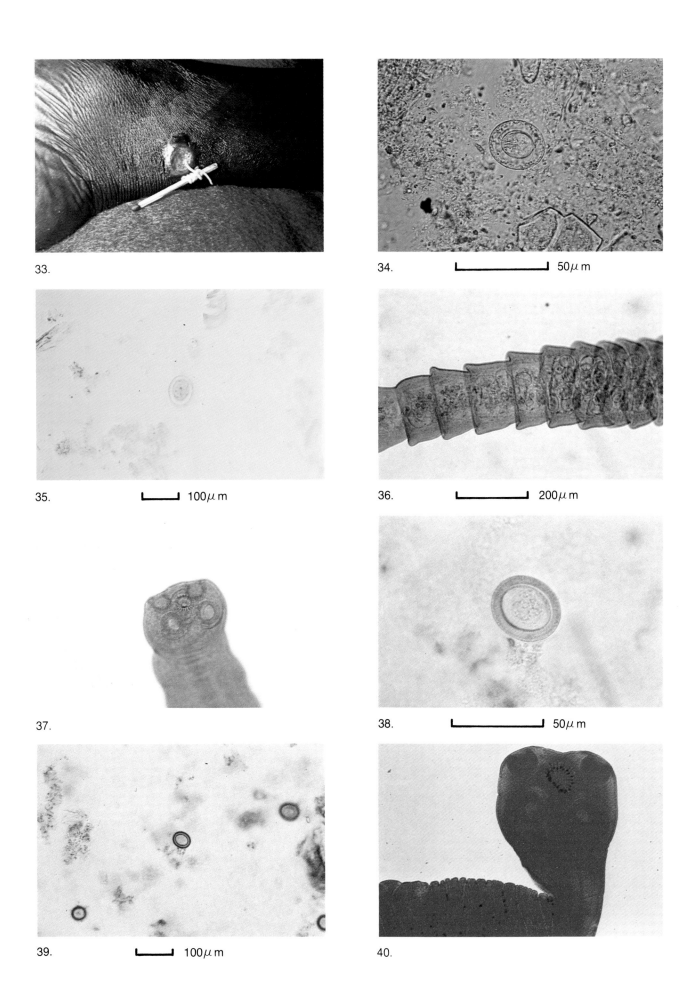

33.

34. ⊢————————⊣ 50μm

35. ⊢————⊣ 100μm

36. ⊢————————⊣ 200μm

37.

38. ⊢————————⊣ 50μm

39. ⊢————⊣ 100μm

40.

41. *Taenia saginata* (beef tapeworm) scolex (100 ×). This is the unarmed tapeworm; the scolex bears only four large, cup-shaped suckers and no hooks.

42. *Taenia solium* gravid proglottid (5 ×). The adult worm measures 2 to 8 meters in length, usually with fewer than 1000 proglottids. The gravid proglottid has 7 to 13 (usually 9) lateral uterine branches (here stained dark brown) filled with eggs, which is diagnostic for the species when recovered in the feces. Gravid proglottids of *Taenia* species must burst open to release eggs because they have no uterine opening. (Note: Handle with care because eggs are infective.)

43. *Taenia saginata* (beef tapeworm) gravid proglottid (5 ×). The adult measures 5 to 10 meters in length and has 1000 to 2000 proglottids. Each gravid proglottid has 15 to 30 lateral uterine branches containing about 80,000 eggs, which is diagnostic for the species when recovered in feces. The life cycle of both worms requires that the eggs be ingested by the appropriate intermediate host (the pig or cow). The eggs hatch in the small intestine after ingestion by the intermediate host, and the six-hooked embryos penetrate the mucosal wall. They are carried by the circulation (blood and lymphatic) to various tissues, where they encyst. Undercooked or raw beef or pork containing *Cysticercus* larvae, when ingested, allow larvae to develop into adults. Toxic metabolites and irritation at the site of scolex attachment in the intestine by adult worms cause the human clinical symptoms. These are variable and frequently vague and include abdominal distress, weight loss, and neuropathies.

44. *Diphyllobothrium latum* (broad fish tapeworm) egg (400 ×). *D. latum* eggs (56 to 76 μm × 40 to 50 μm) are operculated (have a lid) and may be differentiated from operculated eggs of other helminths by the polar knob seen opposite the operculum, the large size, and the undeveloped embryo seen within. Diagnosis is made when these eggs are recovered in stool specimens. Undeveloped eggs discharged from segments of the adult tapeworm must reach fresh water, where they mature and hatch, and the embryo infects the first intermediate host (copepods). Fish ingest infected copepods (water flea) and serve as the second intermediate host. Humans and dogs acquire the infection by eating raw or undercooked parasitized fish containing the infective larval stage, the plerocercoid.

45. *Diphyllobothrium latum* egg (400 ×). The operculum (eggshell cap) of this egg is open. A polar knob is evident at the opposite end of the shell.

46. *Diphyllobothrium latum* egg (100 ×). A low-power view of the same egg.

47. *Diphyllobothrium latem* scolex (5 ×). The scolex of this species does not have hooks or cup-shaped suckers but is characterized by two grooved suckers (bothria), one on each side of the scolex. This worm attaches to the mucosa of the small intestine by the bothria and can grow to 20 meters in length. Eggs develop in cold, clear lakes in temperate regions, including the Great Lakes in North America.

48. *Diphyllobothrium latum* proglottid (10 ×). The mature segment is much wider than it is tall and contains a rosette-shaped uterus. There is a uterine pore through which eggs are discharged. This parasite is found worldwide in areas around fresh water. In the United States, it is found in Florida, the Great Lakes region, and Alaska. The disease is often asymptomatic or is accompanied by vague, digestive disturbances. Some patients develop a macrocytic anemia of the pernicious anemia type because the worm successfully competes with the host for dietary vitamin B_{12} and absorbs it before it can enter the host's circulation. Chains of proglottids may be found in feces.

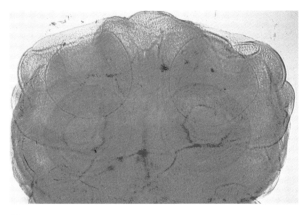

41.

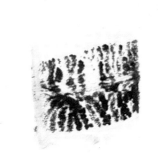

42.

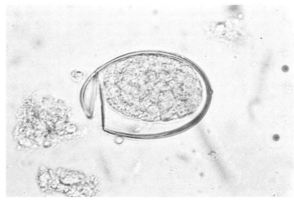

43.

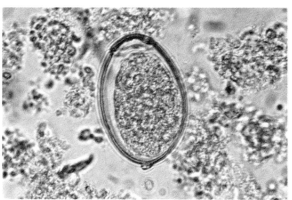

44. |⎯⎯⎯⎯⎯| 50μm

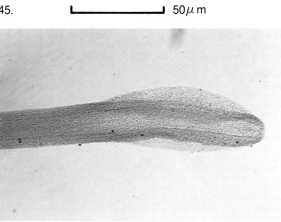

45. |⎯⎯⎯⎯⎯| 50μm

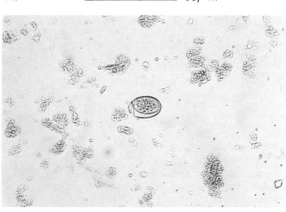

46. |⎯⎯⎯| 100μm

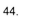

47.

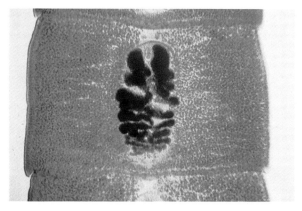

48.

49. *Echinococcus granulosus* (dog tapeworm or hydatid cyst tapeworm) adult (5 ×). This view shows the entire worm, which is 3 to 6 mm long and is found only in the small intestine of the canine host. The dog or wolf is the definitive host and harbors the sexually mature adult parasites. Sheep and other ruminants are natural intermediate hosts and harbor the asexual stage of the parasite in the tissues, but a human can be an accidental intermediate host for *E. granulosus*. Infection of sheep or humans occurs when eggs are ingested in contaminated food or water or by hand-to-mouth transfer from objects soiled with dog feces. Eggs hatch in the small intestine, and larvae migrate to various organs (usually liver or lung) to produce cysts. Dogs and other wild carnivores become infected by eating raw meat containing a hydatid cyst, thus completing the cycle. In humans the produced disease varies with the location of the cyst. There may be no symptoms, or death may result if vital organs are involved. The parasite is found worldwide. Although rare in Europe and most of the United States, except in sheep-raising areas, it is common in Alaska and Canada. Diagnosis in humans is by history of possible exposure; by radiology; by immunodiagnostic skin testing or serologic testing; and by observing hooklets, scolices, and larval cyst membranes in histopathologic sections or other body fluids.

50. *Echinococcus granulosus* (100 ×). A tissue section showing the wall of the hydatid cyst and three brood capsules containing scolices growing into the cyst fluid from germinal tissue that underlies the outer cyst wall.

51. *Echinococcus granulosus* (500 ×). A higher magnification of a single cyst. Each scolex clearly shows the suckers and crown of hooks. Each scolex in a hydatid cyst will grow to an adult tapeworm after ingestion by a dog.

52. *Echinococcus granulosus* cysts. This view shows several small cysts taken from the vertebral column of a patient with spinal cord compression. Cysts in humans can be in any tissue, including bone, but are more common in liver, lung, or central nervous system (CNS).

The Digenea (flukes) are known as flatworms because they appear flat, elongated, and leaf-shaped. Both male and female sex organs are found in each adult fluke that parasitizes the intestine, bile duct, or lungs. The blood flukes (genus *Schistosoma*), however, are unisexual but live paired together in the blood vessels. Attachment is by the oral and ventral cup-shaped suckers; moreover, the tegument of the flukes may bear small spines that aid attachment. These parasites vary in size from less than 1 mm to several centimeters in length. All trematodes require specific species of snail intermediate hosts, and infection of humans occurs either by direct penetration of the skin by a free-swimming cercaria (schistosome species) or by ingestion of an encysted metacercaria (infective larva) of hermaphroditic flukes. Adult flukes live many years.

53. *Fasciola hepatica* (sheep liver fluke) adult (2 ×). This parasite is found in sheep- and cattle-raising areas worldwide, including the United States. Encysted metacercariae on aquatic vegetation, eaten by humans, sheep, or cattle, excyst, burrow through the intestinal wall, migrate to the liver, and work their way through the parenchyma until they enter the proximal bile duct, where they become adults (3 cm × 1.3 cm). Visible structures include the anterior cone, the oral and ventral suckers located at the anterior end, the compact uterus (dark brown) adjacent to the ventral sucker, Mehlis' gland (a round structure centered beneath the uterus), and the testes, occupying the central portion of the fluke. The vitellaria (finely branching, yolk-producing glands) extend from top to bottom toward the outer edges of the parasite and partially cover the testes over the posterior one-third. Disease symptoms reflect traumatic damage, with tissue necrosis and toxic irritation to the liver, bile duct, and gallbladder. Diarrhea, vomiting, irregular fever, jaundice, and eosinophilia are characteristic symptoms.

54. *Fasciola hepatica* egg (400 ×). Diagnosis: by recovery of this large, operculated egg in feces and by clinical signs. This egg is very similar to that of *Fasciolopsis buski* (see Plate 57). Differentiation of eggs of these two parasites is very difficult. Eggs of *F. hepatica* measure 140 μm × 70 μm.

55. *Fasciola hepatica* egg (100 ×). A low-power view of the large *F. hepatica* egg in the midst of naturally occurring fecal debris.

56. *Fasciolopsis buski* (large intestinal fluke) (2 ×). *F. buski* (2 to 7.5 cm × 1 to 2 cm) is found primarily in Asia. Encysted larvae (metacercariae) on vegetation eaten by humans or pigs mature to become adults and attach to the mucosa of the small intestine. Identifiable and differential structures include the unbranched intestinal ceca running laterally from top to bottom toward the outer edges; the two suckers of unequal size (round structures at the top of the organism); the uterus (a dark canal centered under the ventral sucker, branching laterally); Mehlis' gland with attached ovary centered approximately one-third of the way posterior to the ventral sucker; and the testes, branching laterally from the center, beneath the ovary. The anterior end tapers to form the oral sucker, which is visible in this view. Disease symptoms caused by toxic products absorbed into the host's circulation include general edema, diarrhea, vomiting, anorexia, and, possibly, malabsorption syndrome. Slight anemia and eosinophilia occur in severe infections.

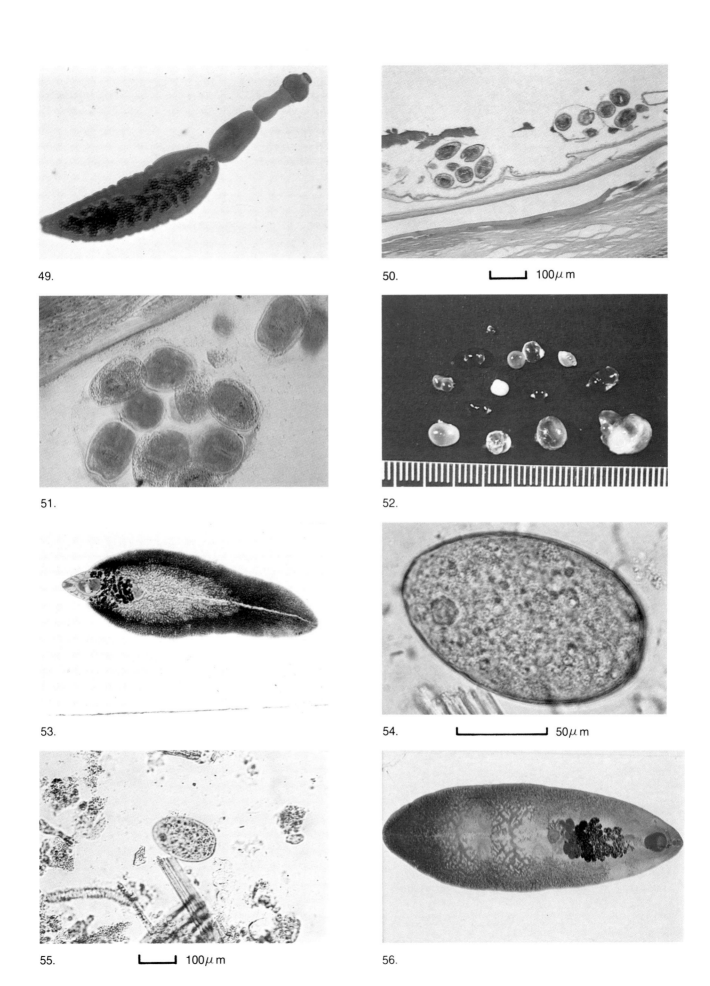

49.

50.　　　　　　　⊢——⊣ 100μm

51.

52.

53.

54.　　　　⊢————⊣ 50μm

55.　　　⊢—⊣ 100μm

56.

57. *Fasciolopsis buski* egg (400 ×). Recovery of this large, thin-shelled, operculated egg (140 μm × 70 μm) is diagnostic. The operculum (lid) is visible here, open at the right end of the egg. This egg is empty; it was previously incubated, and the larva has hatched out of the shell.

58. *Fasciolopsis buski* egg (100 ×). Immediately below this large egg appears a *Trichuris trichiura* egg; this is a very good example of the difference in size between the eggs of the two organisms. The operculum is visible at the left end of the fluke egg, and the material inside of it is yolk. Most of the trematode eggs are undifferentiated when found in fecal specimens. Eggs of all species must reach fresh water before further development occurs. After full development, the first larval form (miracidium) hatches and penetrates the soft tissues of an appropriate intermediate host, the snail. The miracidia develop through several stages to produce free-swimming cercariae, which then (in this species) encyst on aquatic vegetation as metacercariae, which are infective when the vegetation is eaten by a human. *Fasciola hepatica* eggs look identical.

59. *Clonorchis sinensis* (Oriental liver fluke) (4 ×). This adult measures 1 to 2.5 cm × 3 to 5 mm. Humans are infected by eating raw fish, the second intermediate host, containing encysted metacercariae. Larvae excyst in the small intestine and migrate to the bile ducts, where they develop into adult worms. Visible structures include the oral sucker at the anterior end, the ventral sucker one-quarter posteriorly to the oral sucker, the uterus (a dark, branching structure extending downward from the ventral sucker to the ovary), and the testes, immediately below the large, oval Mehlis' gland. The ceca extend from top to bottom toward the outer edge. The vitellaria are parallel to the uterus. This parasite is found throughout the Orient and causes obstructive liver damage with extensive biliary fibrosis. Symptoms result from local irritation and systemic toxemia. Loss of appetite, diarrhea, abdominal pain, and eosinophilia (5 to 40 percent) are common symptoms.

60. *Clonorchis sinensis* egg (500 ×). Eggs (15 μm × 30 μm) are deposited in the bile duct and are evacuated in feces. Diagnosis: recovery of this small, bile-stained egg in feces. Note the thick shell, the characteristic bell shape, and the thickened opercular rim (the shoulders). There is usually a polar knob opposite the operculum.

61. *Clonorchis sinensis* egg (100 ×). A low-power view of a developed *C. sinensis* egg. The eggs are difficult to differentiate from those of other genera (e.g., *Opisthorchis*).

62. *Paragonimus westermani* (lung fluke) (4 ×). This lung-dwelling adult measures 0.8 to 1.2 cm × 4 to 6 mm. Humans are infected by eating raw crab or crayfish, the second intermediate host, containing encysted metacercariae. Larvae excyst in the small intestine; burrow through the mucosa; and migrate through the peritoneal cavity, the diaphragm, and the pleural cavity to the lungs, where they develop into adult worms. Visible structures include the oral sucker at the anterior end; the ovary, which is immediately below the ventral sucker about midway down in the organism; the dark-staining uterus to the left of the ovary; and the testes, located in the clear space beneath the ovary. The branching vitellaria are visible along the outer edges of the parasite. This parasite is found throughout the Orient and parts of Africa. It causes a chronic tuberculosis-type disease with fibrous capsules forming around the adults. Eggs are coughed up in sputum and are visible as orange-brown flecks. Clinical signs resemble those of tuberculosis, including cough with bloody sputum. Adults may invade other organs. Symptoms vary with the location of the adult fluke.

63. *Paragonimus westermani* egg (300 ×). Diagnosis: recovery of this operculated egg (80 to 120 μm × 50 to 60 μm) in sputum or feces. Eggs can be found in fecal specimens when sputum containing eggs is swallowed. Skin testing may provide better evidence of infections than do fecal examinations. Notice the thin shell and the thickened rim around the operculum. The shell also thickens at the end opposite the operculum.

64. *Paragonimus westermani* egg (100 ×). A low-power view of the egg in the center of fecal debris.

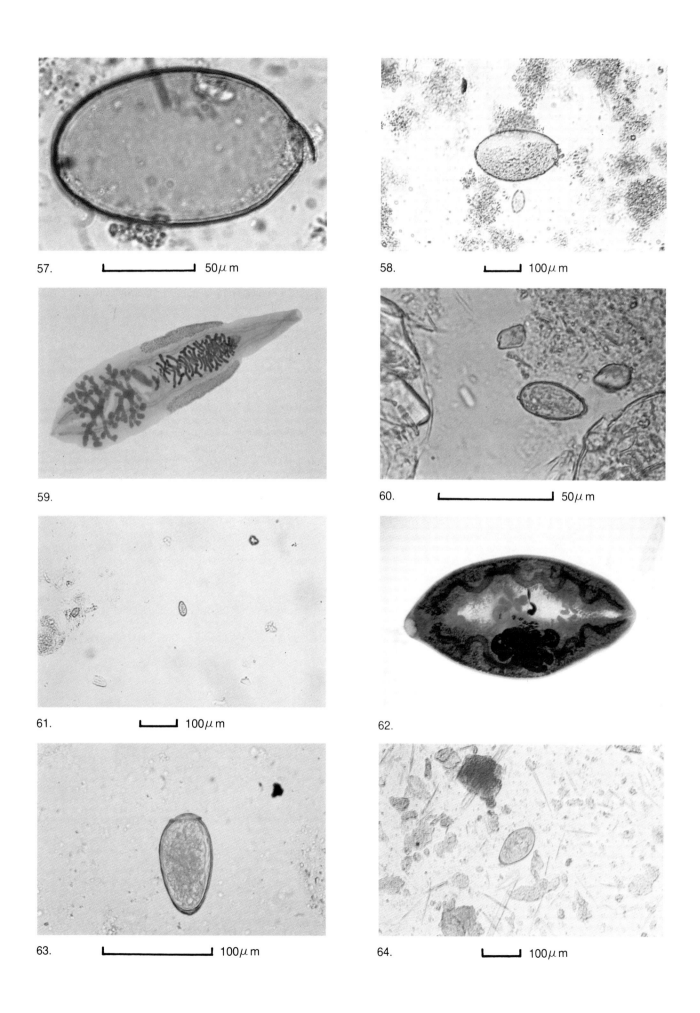

57. |⎯⎯⎯⎯⎯| 50μm

58. |⎯⎯⎯⎯| 100μm

59.

60. |⎯⎯⎯⎯⎯⎯⎯| 50μm

61. |⎯⎯⎯| 100μm

62.

63. |⎯⎯⎯⎯⎯| 100μm

64. |⎯⎯| 100μm

65. *Schistosoma* species (blood flukes). Adults are in copula. The female (15 to 30 mm × 0.2 mm) is seen lying inside the gynecophoral canal of the male. These unisexual worms have a cylindroidal shape and live in pairs, surviving for many years. Infection occurs when free-swimming, fork-tailed cercariae escape from the snail intermediate host; burrow into the capillary bed of feet, legs, or arms of humans; and are carried to the blood vessels of the liver, where they develop into adults. From there, *S. mansoni* and *S. japonicum* migrate to mesenteric veins around the colon. *S. haematobium* migrates to pelvic veins around the urinary bladder.

66. *Schistosoma mansoni* egg (400 ×). Diagnosis: recovery of eggs in feces. Unlike the other trematodes, schistosome eggs do not have an operculum. Note the large size (115 to 175 μm × 50 to 70 μm) and the conspicuous lateral spine protruding from the side near one pole. A ciliated miracidium is indistinct but visible inside this egg, but in fresh specimens it is generally distinct and motile, with active cilia and flame cells. Eggs are deposited into venules, eventually rupture the wall to effect passage into the lumen of the intestine, and are evacuated in the feces. Many eggs are caught in tissues of the liver and intestine, and a granuloma forms around each egg in response to toxic enzymes released by the miracidium. Clinical manifestations include high eosinophilia (up to 50%), gastrointestinal bleeding, rectal polyps, and hepatic cirrhosis. This parasite is found in Africa, the Middle East, parts of South America, the West Indies, and Puerto Rico. Infected persons can frequently be found in immigrant populations living in North American urban centers.

67. *Schistosoma mansoni* egg (100 ×). A low-power view of several eggs. Note the lateral spines on the eggs.

68. *Schistosoma japonicum* egg (400 ×). Diagnosis: recovery of eggs in feces. This egg measures 70 to 100 μm × 50 to 60 μm. A small lateral spine on the eggshell is characteristic for this species. A ciliated miracidium is seen inside the egg. The produced disease is similar to that of *S. mansoni*. Because *S. japonicum* produces 10 times as many eggs as *S. mansoni*, the disease is more severe. Many eggs are swept back into the bloodstream to the liver and are trapped, causing fibrosis and cirrhosis of the liver. Toxic symptoms are severe. This parasite is found in the Orient.

69. *Schistosoma japonicum* eggs (100 ×). A low-power view of several eggs. The lateral spine is barely visible in some eggs. *S. mekongi* eggs are similar but small (50 to 75 μm × 40 to 65 μm). These eggs are often coated with fecal debris and are more difficult to notice.

70. *Schistosoma haematobium* egg (400 ×). Diagnosis: recovery of eggs in urine. This egg measures 115 to 175 μm × 40 to 70 μm. A pointed terminal spine is characteristic for this species. A ciliated miracidium is visible inside. Egg deposition by *S. haematobium* causes local traumatic damage to the rectum and the urinary bladder. Bladder colic is a cardinal symptom. Blood, pus cells, and necrotic tissue debris are passed during urination. Systemic symptoms are less severe than those produced by the other schistosomes. There is a high correlation with bladder cancer in infected persons. This parasite is found in Africa, the Middle East, and Portugal.

71. *Schistosoma haematobium* egg (300 ×). A high-power view of the egg, showing a differently shaped terminal spine. Urine should be concentrated to aid detection. Eggs are most often in the last few drops expelled from the bladder.

Amebae are unicellular protozoa, some of which may be parasitic in humans. These organisms are found worldwide, and some can live as parasitic or commensal trophozoites (the motile, feeding, reproductive stage) in the lower gastrointestinal tract of humans. Most intestinal protozoa form a cyst stage (a dormant, protective stage for the parasite in unfavorable environments after being evacuated in the host's feces) and in the cyst form may remain viable for long periods in warm, moist conditions. Transmission of intestinal amebic diseases is from ingested cysts in fecally contaminated food, soil, or water. Cysts are most commonly passed in feces by asymptomatic carriers.

72. *Entamoeba histolytica* trophozoite (10 to 60 μm) (1000 ×). This ameba is pathogenic for humans. It can invade the intestinal mucosa, causing flask-shaped lesions and bloody diarrhea. The trophozoite releases lytic enzymes and can also spread to other tissues, such as the liver, and cause amebic ulceration. Notice the nucleus, which has a light chromatin ring at the edges, surrounding a centrally located karyosome (compare with *E. coli*, Plate 78). The cytoplasm is finely granular as compared with that of *E. coli*. This is a trichrome-stained organism.

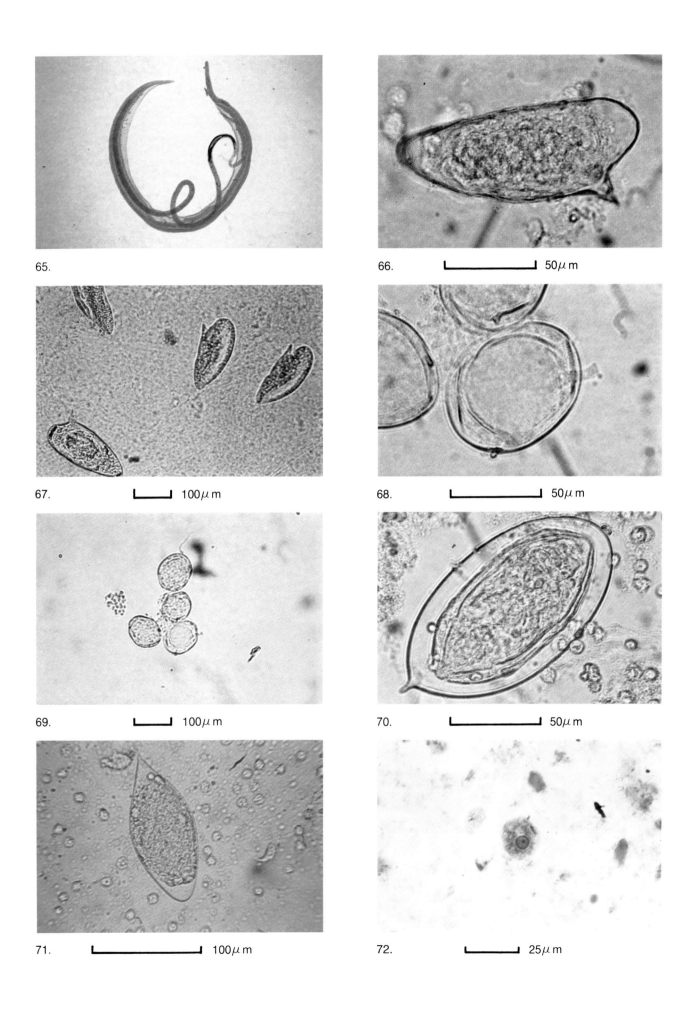

65.

66.   ⊢━━━━━━━┥ 50μm

67.   ⊢━━━┥ 100μm

68.   ⊢━━━━━━━┥ 50μm

69.   ⊢━━━┥ 100μm

70.   ⊢━━━━━━━┥ 50μm

71.   ⊢━━━━━━━━━┥ 100μm

72.   ⊢━━━┥ 25μm

73. *Entamoeba histolytica* (1000 ×). This trophozoite in feces contains five engulfed red blood cells, the presence of which is a diagnostic feature, inasmuch as no other ameba will contain these. In saline solution, the trophozoite will exhibit progressive, active motility, with thin, fingerlike pseudopodia.

74. *Entamoeba histolytica* cyst (1000 ×). Cysts of *E. histolytica* are over 10 μm in size (10 to 20 μm). There are up to four typical nuclei in the mature cyst. One nucleus is clearly visible here. The nuclear structure is identical in both trophozoites and cysts. The dark bars are chromatoid bodies, generally cigar-shaped, which may be found in cysts. These are crystalline RNA. Iron hematoxylin stain.

75. *Entamoeba histolytica* cyst (1000 ×) showing four nuclei. Iodine stain.

76. *Entamoeba hartmanni* trophozoite (1000 ×). Note the morphologic similarity between the nucleus of this commensal and that in Plate 72. This organism was previously identified as *E. histolytica* but is now known as *E. hartmanni*. It is not pathogenic but morphologically resembles *E. histolytica*, differing only in size; it is less than 10 μm in size. This characteristic is important because correct diagnosis depends upon the careful measurement of the parasite. A trophozoite or cyst resembling *E. histolytica* that is less than 10 μm in diameter is classified as *E. hartmanni*.

77. *Entamoeba hartmanni* cyst (1000 ×). The cyst (5 to 10 μm) resembles that of *E. histolytica* but is classified as *E. hartmanni* because of its small size, the upper limits being 10 μm. This cyst is stained with iodine. It can have up to four nuclei. It is important to differentiate *E. histolytica* from this and other nonpathogenic amebae to ensure correct treatment of the patient.

78. *Entamoeba coli* trophozoite (1000 ×). This is a common commensal, and care must be taken to differentiate it from *E. histolytica*. Notice the nucleus, which has a dark, irregularly thickened chromatin ring around the membrane and a large, eccentrically located karyosome. This parasite is often larger than *E. histolytica* (15 to 60 μm) and has coarser cytoplasm and sluggish motility, with blunt pseudopodia.

79. *Entamoeba coli* trophozoite (1000 ×). This trophozoite has a very large karyosome located next to the chromatin ring.

80. *Entamoeba coli* cyst (1000 ×). Five nuclei are visible in the cyst (10 to 30 μm). *E. coli* is differentiated from *E. histolytica* by the nuclear morphology and by the fact that the cyst may contain up to eight nuclei, rather than four. Chromatoid bars in stained cysts will be splinterlike, with pointed ends.

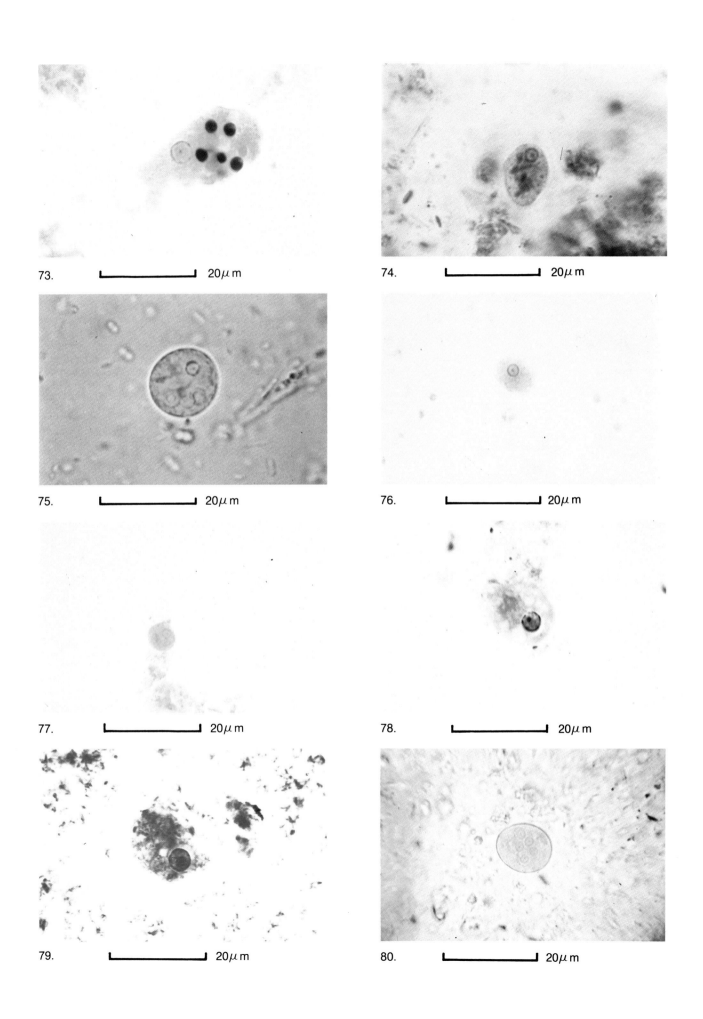

73.   20μm   74.   20μm

75.   20μm   76.   20μm

77.   20μm   78.   20μm

79.   20μm   80.   20μm

81. *Entamoeba coli* cysts (100 ×). A low-power view of several cysts. One is seen at the center of the field, and several others are evident in the lower left area, all appearing as dark dots. This view demonstrates the importance of scanning a part of all fecal slides under high power so that protozoa are not missed. These cysts also should be examined at even higher magnifications to see the nuclei and other features for correct diagnosis of the parasite species.

82. *Endolimax nana* trophozoite (1000 ×). Note the large karyosome in the nucleus. The fine chromatin ring is not usually visible. This feature is diagnostic for this commensal (6 to 12 μm). Note also the cytoplasmic vacuoles.

83. *Endolimax nana* cyst (2000 ×). The ovoid mature cyst has four nuclei. Note the large karyosome (dark dots). The chromatin ring is not visible. These features are diagnostic. This parasite (8 to 10 μm) may be confused with *E. histolytica* if care is not taken when examining the nuclear structure and the cyst shape.

84. *Iodamoeba bütschlii* trophozoite (1000 ×). Note the large karyosome and light chromatin ring in the nucleus of the organism (12 to 15 μm). The cytoplasm is coarsely granular, and a small, light vacuole that contains glycogen is visible.

85. *Iodamoeba bütschlii* cyst (1000 ×). Note the large karyosome in the single nucleus of this trichrome-stained cyst (5 to 20 μm). A large vacuole from which glycogen has been removed by the staining process is visible (clear area inside cyst), which is diagnostic for this commensal. The glycogen vacuole stains dark brown when an iodine wet mount is used. The nucleus of this species does not stain with iodine.

Flagellates are unicellular protozoa that move by means of flagella (motile fibrils extending from the body of the organism). Many of the flagellates have a trophozoite stage, which is the active, feeding, motile form, and also a cyst stage, which is a dormant, protective stage for the parasite in unfavorable environments outside the host's intestine. Transmission of the intestinal flagellates is by ingestion of fecally contaminated food or drink; *Trichomonas vaginalis* trophozoites are directly transmitted during sexual intercourse; and the hemoflagellates (found in the blood or tissues) are transmitted by arthropod intermediate hosts.

86. *Dientamoeba fragilis* trophozoite (1000 ×). This flagellate (5 to 12 μm) does not form cysts. Note that it has two nuclei. This feature is diagnostic inasmuch as no other ameboid trophozoite has more than one nucleus. This organism may be pathogenic and may cause diarrhea in humans.

87. *Giardia lamblia* trophozoites (1000 ×). These flagellates (10 to 20 μm × 15 μm) live in the duodenum and often do not produce disease. When present in large numbers, they may cause epigastric pain and diarrhea. Note the smiling face–like appearance of the trophozoite, which is bilaterally symmetric with two anterior nuclei, a central axostyle, and four pairs of flagella. In fresh fecal wet-mount preparations, the motile trophozoite moves like a leaf falling from a tree.

88. *Giardia lamblia* cyst (1000 ×). Diagnosis: recovery of trophozoites or cysts (8 μm × 10 μm) in feces. The mature cyst has four nuclei, although the immature cyst may have only two. Three are visible in the upper cyst in this view.

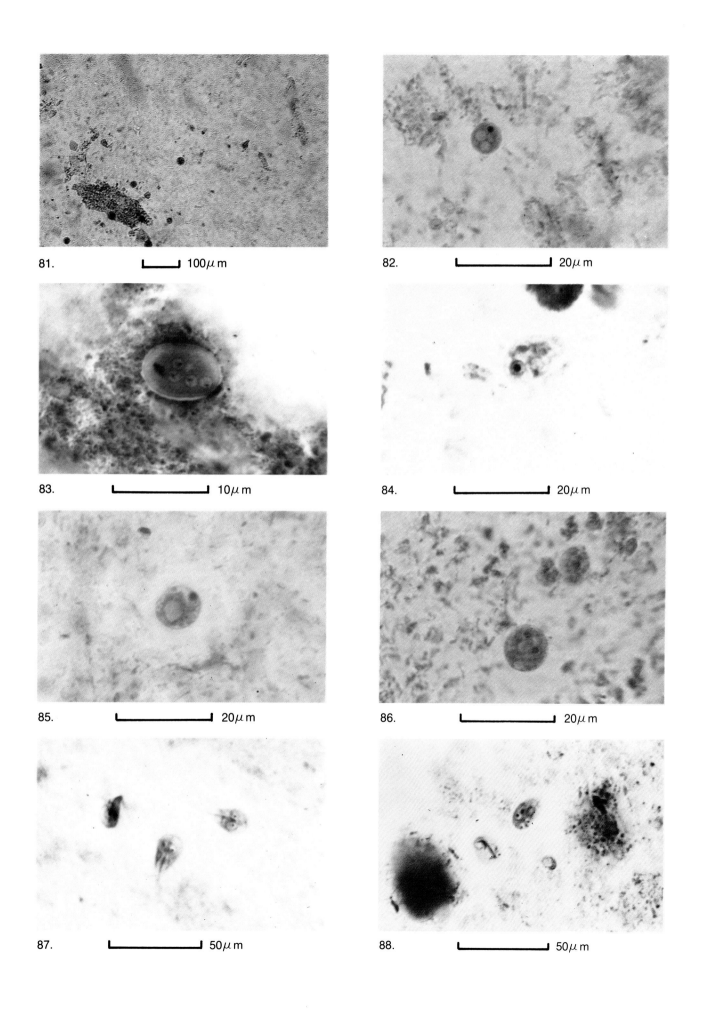

81. ├───┤ 100μm

82. ├───┤ 20μm

83. ├───┤ 10μm

84. ├───┤ 20μm

85. ├───┤ 20μm

86. ├───┤ 20μm

87. ├───┤ 50μm

88. ├───┤ 50μm

89. Unusual sight of *Entamoeba coli* trophozoite containing several ingested *Giardia lamblia* cysts (1000 ×).

90. *Giardia lamblia* trophozoites (1000 ×). This stained section of duodenal mucosa shows two trophozoites adhering. Note the two nuclei visible in the trophozoite centered in the field.

91. *Chilomastix mesnili* trophozoite (1000 ×). This commensal flagellate (7 μm × 20 μm) lives in the upper large intestine and does not produce disease. Note the single prominent nucleus at the rounded anterior end. The posterior is tapered with a noticeably angled projection. There are four anterior flagella and a distinct longitudinal spiral groove. Viable trophozoites move in a spiral path.

92. *Chilomastix mesnili* cyst (1000 ×). Diagnosis: recovery of cysts (5 μm × 8 μm) in feces. There is a single, large nucleus in this lemon-shaped cyst. Correct diagnosis is important so that this is not confused with *Giardia* or other pathogenic infection.

93. *Trichomonas vaginalis* trophozoite (1000 ×). This parasite (18 μm × 25 μm) is recovered in urine or in urethral or vaginal mucosal scrapings. Symptoms in women vary from mild irritation to painful itching, with a frothy, yellowish vaginal discharge. Infected men are usually asymptomatic carriers. There are four anterior flagella, a large nucleus, and an undulating membrane (not visible in this view) extending along one-half of the body. *T. vaginalis* appears slightly larger than leukocytes, and the whipping motion of the flagella is clearly visible in fresh, unstained urine. *Trichomonas* species do not form cysts. *T. hominis* is a nonpathogenic intestinal flagellate found in feces; *T. gingivalis* trophozoite may be found in the mouth and is also nonpathogenic.

Two genera of flagellates are found as parasites of blood and tissue in humans. The *Leishmania* parasites have two forms in their life cycle: the amastigote form, which multiplies in macrophages in humans, and the promastigote form found in the midgut of the sandfly, *Phlebotomus* spp. (the intermediate host). The other bloodborne genus parasitic in humans is *Trypanosoma*. These organisms are in trypomastigote form in the bloodstream and other tissues in humans, and in the epimastigote form in the arthropod intermediate host (except for *T. cruzi*, which is also seen as the amastigote form in human heart muscle).

94. Amastigote form (1000 ×). Many amastigotes (3 μm to 5 μm in diameter) are seen in this view. The nucleus and the smaller, bar-shaped kinetoplast are visible in each organism as seen in the center of this field. The leishmania invade reticuloendothelial cells and macrophages of humans. The disease produced by the organisms of each species is as follows:

1. *L. tropica* (Old World leishmaniasis). Local lesions occur at the site of the sandfly bite, followed by focal necrosis. Although it may be complicated by secondary bacterial infection, the disease is usually self-limiting and produces life-long immunity to reinfection. This parasite is found in Africa, India, and the Middle East.
2. *L. braziliensis* (New World leishmaniasis). The primary lesion is local, as with *L. tropica*, but the ulcer heals slowly. Erosion of soft tissues, especially of the nose, mouth, ears, and cheeks, often occurs years later, inasmuch as this organism tends to migrate to secondary sites, often complicated by bacterial invasion followed by local and systemic symptoms. This parasite is found in Central and South America.
3. *L. donovani* (kala-azar). The local primary lesion is usually not reported. The amastigotes gain access to the bloodstream or lymphatics and eventually spread to fixed tissue macrophages in the viscera. Sites of this invasion are the liver, spleen, and bone marrow, where multiplication usually proceeds unchecked. Anemia usually follows because of increased production of macrophages and decreased erythropoietic activity. The acute phase of the systemic disease is characterized by double spiking fever fluctuating daily (between 90°F and 104°F). There is moderate erythrocytopenia, absolute monocytosis, and neutropenia. Massive hepatosplenomegaly occurs because of parasite multiplication, and death frequently occurs if the patient is untreated. This parasite is widely distributed, except in the United States.

95. *Leishmania donovani* (1000 ×) seen multiplying in a macrophage in a press preparation of spleen tissue.

96. Leishmaniasis. A typical skin lesion caused by *L. braziliensis*. Note the open ulcer on the man's forehead.

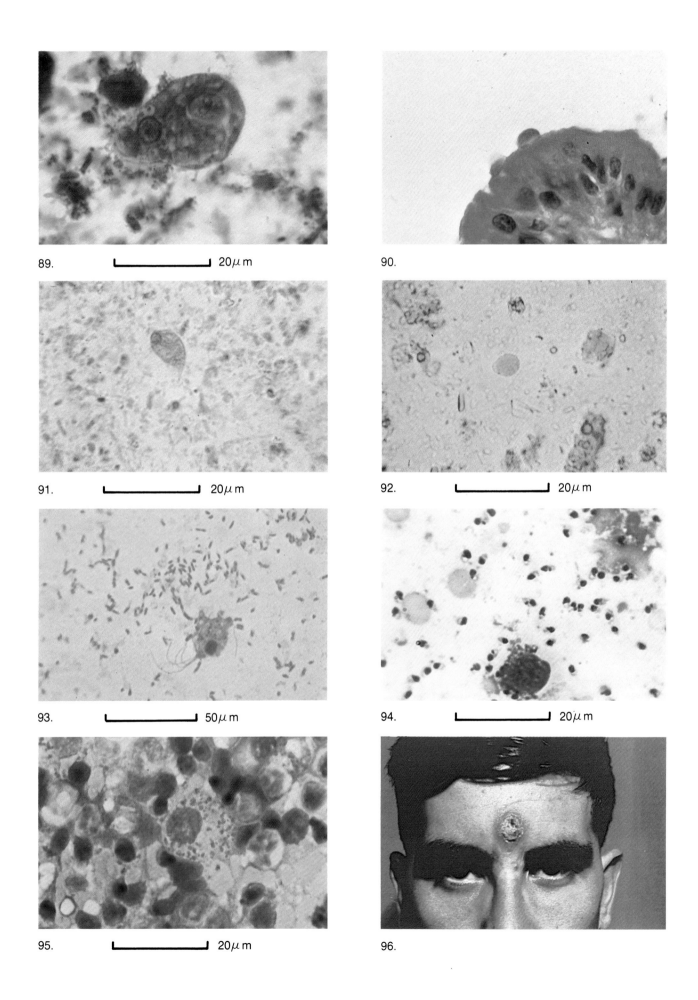

89.   ⊢━━━━━━━┥ 20μm

90.

91.   ⊢━━━━━┥ 20μm

92.   ⊢━━━━━┥ 20μm

93.   ⊢━━━━━┥ 50μm

94.   ⊢━━━━━┥ 20μm

95.   ⊢━━━━━┥ 20μm

96.

97. Promastigote form (100 ×). This stage is found in the midgut and proboscis of the sandfly, *Phlebotomus.* It is the infective form of leishmaniasis and is transferred to humans by the biting fly. The large nucleus, bar-shaped kinetoplast, and flagellum are visible. Note the relative position of these structures.

98. Trypomastigote form (1000 ×). The trypanosome is found extracellularly, free in the blood. It is the infective form transferred to humans by the biting arthropod vector (intermediate host). Trypanosome species are not readily differentiated in peripheral blood. Visible structures include the flagellum, the large central nucleus, and the undulating membrane that is attached to the kinetoplast at the posterior end of the organism. The diseases produced by these organisms are as follows:

1. The sleeping sickness diseases produced by *T. rhodesiense* and *T. gambiense* are similar, differing primarily in the severity of the second stage, which is so severe with *T. rhodesiense* infections that death rapidly results. The disease begins with local inflammation at the site of the fly bite (tsetse fly). This subsides as the trypanosomes enter the blood. They migrate to the lymph nodes, where severe inflammation occurs because of rapid multiplication. Toxic metabolites and occlusion of vascular sinuses by the proliferating organisms may cause death at this stage. Enlarged lymph nodes, myocarditis, fever episodes, edema, and rapid weight loss are cardinal symptoms for *T. rhodesiense*. Trypanosomes invade the central nervous system in the third stage to produce sleeping sickness and eventually death. *T. gambiense* usually proceeds to this stage. The posterior cervical lymph nodes in the neck are invaded and undergo massive swelling. This is called Winterbottom's sign. Other nodes may be invaded, producing weakness, pain, and cramps.
2. *T. cruzi* (Chagas' disease). The primary lesion at the bite site of the reduviid bug intermediate host is often near the eye, producing unilateral edema of the eyelid (Romaña's sign). Next, primary parasitemia with S- or C-shaped trypanosomes with a large kinetoplast (as seen in this view) occurs in the blood, causing fever and toxic conditions resembling typhoid fever (may be fatal in children). The chronic disease is characterized by leishmanial forms multiplying in tissue macrophages, and symptoms of tissue invasion, including enlargement of the spleen, occur. Cardiac and central nervous system pathology occurs as tissue destruction continues. There may be fever episodes and parasitemia when trypanosomes are free in the blood.

Diagnosis of these diseases is confirmed when parasites are recovered in blood or seen in tissue specimens. Trypanosomes are 15 to 30 μm in length.

99. *Trypanosoma cruzi* (amastigote form) in cardiac tissue (1000 ×). The trypomastigote in reduviid bug feces is pushed into the bite wound when the host scratches at the bite site, and these circulate in the blood until phagocytized, or they invade tissue macrophages, after which they change to the amastigote form. Note the nest of multiplying amastigote forms in the heart muscle. Trypomastigote forms can be found in blood.

The Ciliata

100. *Balantidium coli* trophozoite (400 ×). This organism (40 μm × 60 μm) is a ciliate that is characterized by having many short cilia on the surface of both the motile and encysted trophozoite. *B. coli* is the only ciliate pathogenic for humans. The disease is characterized by invasion of the intestinal submucosa with inflammation and ulcer formation. There may be fulminating diarrhea in heavy infections or an asymptomatic carrier state in light infections. This organism has two nuclei: a large, kidney bean–shaped macronucleus and a small, round micronucleus not visible in this view.

101. *Balantidium coli* cyst (400 ×). This large, round cyst (50 μm) is characterized by the presence of macronuclei and micronuclei; the latter are rarely seen, but when present, generally appear as small dots near the concavity of the macronucleus. Cilia are evident around the inside edge of the cyst on the organism. This form, or the trophozoite, is diagnostic when recovered in feces or seen in intestinal tissue.

102. *Balantidium coli* cyst (100 ×). A low-power view of the cyst. This large parasite is easily recognized even at this magnification.

Sporozoa are protozoa that have both a sexual and an asexual phase in their life cycle. The genus *Plasmodium* includes the malaria parasites. The asexual phase is found in the human intermediate host, and the sexual phase occurs in the definitive host, the *Anopheles* mosquito. Sporozoites are injected into the blood by the biting mosquito and then invade liver cells. The asexual stages of malaria first multiply in the liver and later in peripheral blood. Asexual schizogony results in release of merozoites that either may invade new red blood cells and develop into new schizonts or develop to become male and female gametocytes. If the mosquito ingests gametocytes while feeding, these will develop throughout the sexual cycle to produce new sporozoites, the infective form for humans. The clinical symptoms vary with the species of parasite, but all cause anemia (because of destruction of the red blood cells by the schizont form), headaches, general weakness, and a characteristic repetitive fever and chills syndrome.

103. *Plasmodium vivax* (benign tertian malaria). This drawing shows the erythrocytic stages of *P. vivax*. The prominent feature is the presence of Schüffner's dots. These appear as red spots on infected red blood cells on a stained blood smear and are seen in all developmental stages after the early trophozoite stage. The infected red blood cell is larger than normal red blood cells because the parasites preferentially invade reticulocytes, the larger, immature blood cell. The trophozoite divides to form a schizont containing 16 to 18 merozoites, which is a differentiating characteristic for *P. vivax*.

104. *Plasmodium vivax* (100 ×). A trophozoite is clearly visible in the center of the field. Note the red Schüffner's dots. Note also the ring (blue) and the chromatin dot (red) of the trophozoite. Each ring form (about one-third of the cell diameter in size) represents one parasite; multiple parasites in a red cell are not commonly seen in this species.

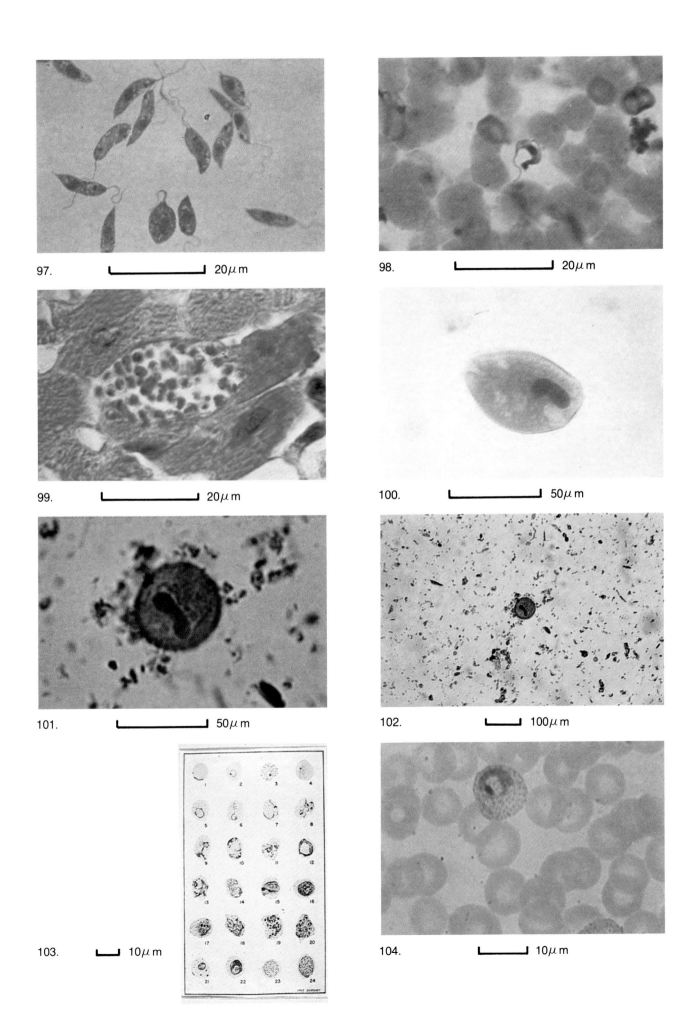

97. |⎣_____⎦| 20μm

98. |⎣_____⎦| 20μm

99. |⎣_____⎦| 20μm

100. |⎣_____⎦| 50μm

101. |⎣_____⎦| 50μm

102. |⎣_____⎦| 100μm

103. |⎣__⎦| 10μm

104. |⎣__⎦| 10μm

105. *Plasmodium vivax* (1000 ×). An older trophozoite than that in the previous plate is seen in the center of the field. Note the larger size of the red cell, the bizarre ameboid shape of the motile trophozoite, and the characteristic Schüffner's dots.

106. *Plasmodium vivax* (1000 ×). An older trophozoite than that in the previous plate is shown. This cell is enlarged and Schüffner's dots are evident. The trophozoite is clearly ameboid in its movements. Plates 104 to 109 clearly illustrate the maturation of the trophozoite stage of *P. vivax*.

107. *Plasmodium vivax* (1000 ×). Developing schizont. Many merozoites are seen inside the cell. A trophozoite appears in the upper right of the field.

108. *Plasmodium vivax* (1000 ×). Mature schizont. Fourteen merozoites are visible inside the cell. Characteristically, the schizont divides to form 16 to 18 merozoites. Development from the invasion of the red blood cell by the trophozoite to the fully mature schizont occurs in 48 hours.

109. *Plasmodium vivax* (1000 ×). Mature schizont. Eighteen merozoites are visible inside the cell. The red blood cell ruptures, releasing the merozoites, which may invade new red blood cells to repeat the asexual erythrocytic cycle. Some merozoites invade red cells and become male or female gametocytes, which are part of the sexual cycle in the mosquito after the gametocytes are ingested in a blood meal.

110. *Plasmodium ovale*. This view shows the erythrocytic stages of *P. ovale*. The red blood cells are enlarged and oval in shape. This parasite is rare in humans and may be confused with *P. malariae* when Schüffner's dots are not present or with *P. vivax* when Schüffner's dots are present.

111, 112. *Plasmodium ovale* trophozoites (1000 ×). This parasite is similar to *P. vivax* because Schüffner's dots are visible. It also resembles *P. malariae* because the mature schizont usually contains 8 to 12 merozoites. The diagnostic characteristic, when present, is the ragged, irregular appearance and oval shape of the host red blood cell, as can be seen here.

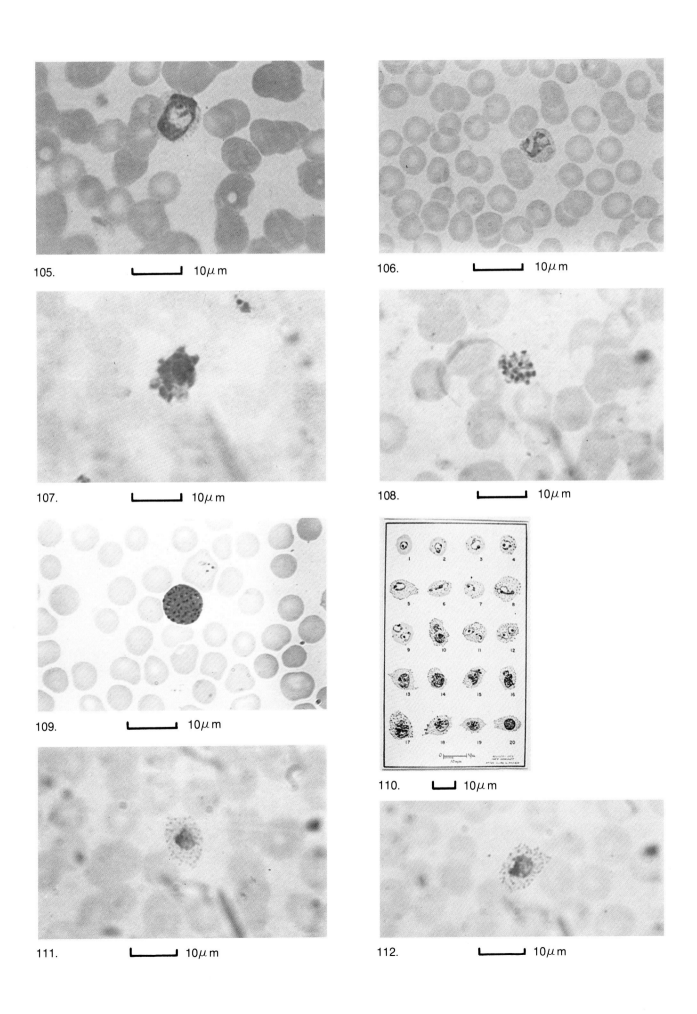

105.   10μm

106.   10μm

107.   10μm

108.   10μm

109.   10μm

110.   10μm

111.   10μm

112.   10μm

113. *Plasmodium malariae* (quartan malaria). This view depicts erythrocytic stages of *P. malariae*. The trophozoite measures about one-third of the diameter of the red blood cell. The prominent features include a large ring form; the band form of the early schizont with coarse, dark granules; and the mature schizont, containing 8 to 12 merozoites, assuming a characteristic rosette shape with malaria pigment deposited in the center of the rosette.

114. *Plasmodium malariae* trophozoite (1000 ×). The band-form trophozoite across the red cell is characteristic during the early development of the schizont.

115. *Plasmodium malariae* schizont (1000 ×). A schizont containing seven merozoites is seen in the upper left corner. By 72 hours after the trophozoite enters the red blood cell, the mature form contains 8 to 10 merozoites and assumes the characteristic rosette shape. Two young trophozoites are also seen in this view.

116. *Plasmodium malariae* gametocyte (1000 ×). This form is similar to that of *P. vivax* but is smaller and contains less pigment.

117. *Plasmodium falciparum* (malignant subtertian malaria). This plate demonstrates the erythrocytic stages of *P. falciparum*. The prominent features are small ring forms with double chromatin dots, multiple rings in the same cell, and crescent-shaped gametocytes. Other stages in schizont formation are not seen in peripheral blood because these (other) stages of maturation occur in the capillaries of internal organs.

118. *Plasmodium falciparum* ring forms (1000 ×). Note the small ring size and multiple infections, not seen with *P. vivax* or *P. malariae*.

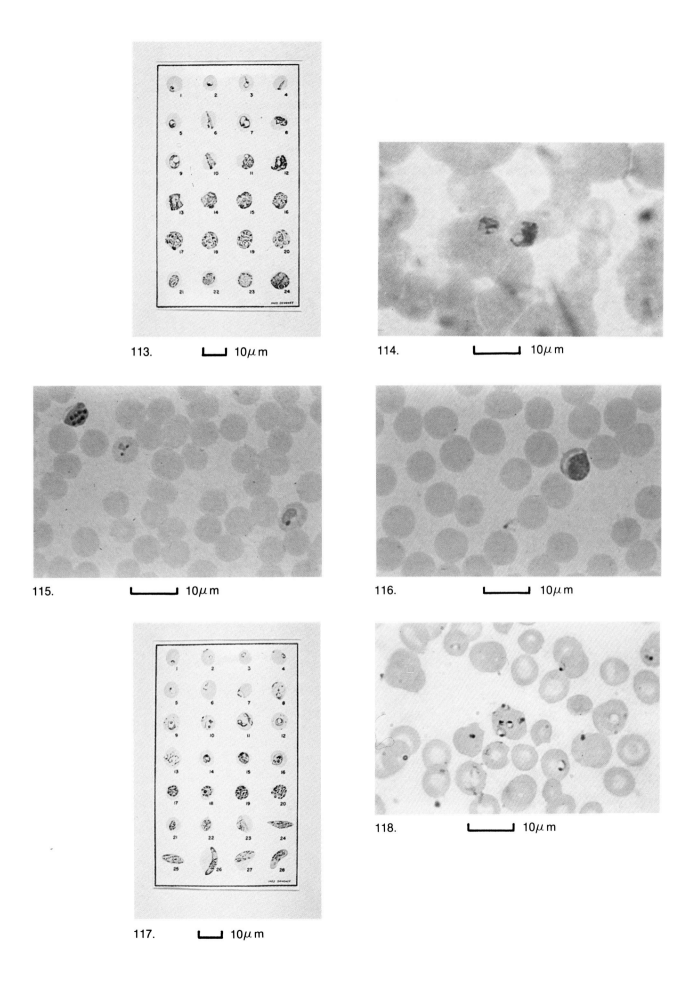

113. |___| 10μm

114. |___| 10μm

115. |___| 10μm

116. |___| 10μm

117. |___| 10μm

118. |___| 10μm

119. Double malaria infection (1000 ×). A *P. vivax* trophozoite is shown in the center of the field. The small ring form seen at upper left has a double chromatin dot, a diagnostic feature of *P. falciparum* rings.

120. *Plasmodium falciparum* gametocyte (1000 ×). Note the characteristic crescent or banana shape of this form.

Malaria has been found worldwide, but control measures have essentially eliminated the disease from many countries, including the United States. It is still a major problem in Africa, Asia, Central and South America, and the South Pacific. Diagnosis: clinical signs and observation of the parasite in thick and thin blood films obtained ideally during the fever cycle. Other important sporozoan parasites are noted below.

121. *Toxoplasma gondii* trophozoites (1000 ×). *T. gondii* trophozoites viewed by fluorescence microscopy in the indirect fluorescent antibody test (IFAT). This is a negative test result, indicating that patient's serum, previously incubated with these organisms, has no detectable antibody to *T. gondii.* No green fluorescence is observable.

122. *Toxoplasma gondii* trophozoites (1000 ×). This is a positive IFAT result for the detection of antibodies to *T. gondii* in serum. Note the green fluorescence over the entire body of the organisms, indicating the presence of antibodies bound to the surface.

123. *Toxoplasma* pseudocyst (400 ×). A dormant pseudocyst filled with bradyzoites of *T. gondii* as seen in a brain section. Immunosuppression of the host would allow these trophozoites to emerge and successfully invade new host cells and to continue multiplication. Brain pseudocysts are also infective if ingested by the definitive host (cats) from mouse brains.

124. *Sarcocystis* spp. (1000 ×). A stained section of muscle tissue in which one can see a sarcocyst filled with potentially infective organisms. These are infective if ingested by the definitive host.

125. *Pneumocystis carinii* (1000 ×). A Romanovsky-stained lung touch preparation. Note the cystlike structure in the center, which contains eight parasites.

126. *Pneumocystis carinii* (400 ×). A methenamine silver stain of lung tissue. Note the darkly stained cyst wall of the parasites within the honeycomb material in the alveolar spaces.

Color Plate Credits
Clay Adams: 1, 6, 9, 13, 15, 24, 26, 27, 29, 32, 41, 48, 51, 59, 60, 67, 75, 86, 89, 91, 93, 97, 104, 105.
David M. Wright, M.D.: 90, 95, 123, 124.
Herman Zaiman, M.D.: 3, 4, 5, 12, 19, 23, 28, 30, 31, 33, 40, 42, 43, 49, 52, 72, 79, 83, 88, 94, 96, 99, 106, 109, 115, 116, 118, 125, 126.
Centers for Disease Control: 25, 73, 76, 77, 78, 80, 84, 87, 92.
National Institutes of Health: 103, 110, 113, 117.

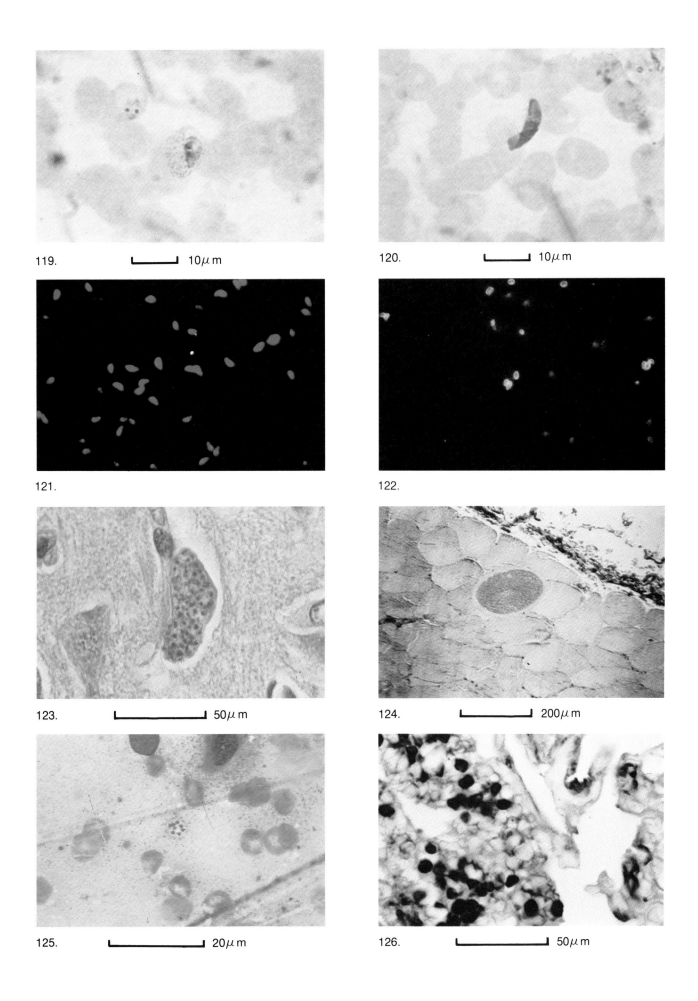

119.   ⊢————⊣ 10μm

120.   ⊢————⊣ 10μm

121.

122.

123.   ⊢————⊣ 50μm

124.   ⊢————⊣ 200μm

125.   ⊢————⊣ 20μm

126.   ⊢————⊣ 50μm

CHAPTER 1

Introduction

North Americans do not suffer from a multitude of harmful parasites largely because of general good health; high standards of education, nutrition, and sanitation; a temperate climate; and the absence of necessary **vectors**. Parasitic infections do exist in this country, however, and are still far from eradicated. Increased travel throughout the world and the general low level of understanding about parasitic infections have added to the problem of disease transmission in the United States. Many other parts of the world have levels of parasite-induced morbidity and mortality among humans and animals as well as parasitic damage to crops that are great drains on manpower and food productivity, thus affecting the international economy. In recognizing this problem, the World Health Organization (WHO) named five parasitic diseases* as among the six most harmful infective diseases afflicting humanity today. More than 1 billion people are afflicted with parasites.

To prepare you to identify organisms that parasitize humans, this book explains parasitism as a biologic concept and introduces specific parasites of medical importance, including the information necessary to assist in the diagnosis of infection. The life cycles of parasites of major medical importance are displayed graphically and pictorially to help you understand how transmission and control of the spread of infection can occur and also how the location of each parasite stage in the human body correlates with clinical symptoms and pathology. Additionally, knowing the life cycle helps you to understand which parasite stage will be seen in body specimens, such as blood, urine, feces, or sputum; this is the key to diagnosis. For substantive review of any particular parasite, you are referred to a variety of texts and specific journal articles in the bibliography of each chapter. Throughout the text you will find words in bold type (e.g., **vector**) that are defined in the glossary of each chapter; a medical dictionary, however, will be helpful to you in your studies. Pertinent references, both classical and up-to-date, have been included in the bibliography to guide you toward in-depth studies in various areas of parasitology, such as the biochemistry, treatment, pathology, or immunology of parasitic infections. This text is best used in conjunction with a course that includes supplementary laboratory experiences. This text presents the multicellular parasites first, because the stages of these parasites, which are generally readily observable under magnification, are relatively easy to find and identify. By the time you have worked through the multicellular parasites, practice with microscopic and other techniques will have made you more effective and efficient in locating and identifying the protozoa and differentiating them from other formed, unicellular structures or artifacts. Treatment (drug or other treatment recommended) is also included for each organism infecting humans. New regulatory requirements related to reagent and specimen handling, as well as new findings and classifications of parasites, have mandated a new edition of this text.

---

*Malaria, leishmaniasis, trypanosomiasis, onchocerciasis, and schistosomiasis.

In order to function as a competent parasitologist, prepared to aid in accurate diagnosis of parasitic infections, you must exhibit knowledge and skills in both clinical and academic areas. This self-study text is designed to help you reach that goal. In addition to chapter presentations of each parasite, an extensive descriptive key accompanying the color photographs is located at the front of the book. These have been carefully chosen to provide a complete depiction of each parasite under discussion. The photographs and descriptive key are arranged in the same sequence as the species presented in the text and should be studied after you have studied the appropriate chapter.

The pre-test in this section is designed to allow you to evaluate your general knowledge of medical parasitology. Following each chapter, a brief post-test enables you to judge your mastery of that particular area. Learning objectives at the beginning of each chapter should guide your study. Review each chapter and plate key until you have completed your learning tasks as determined by a successful challenge of the post-test. A final examination at the end of the text allows you to evaluate your self-paced learning accomplishment. Answer keys for all tests are at the back of the book. A score of 80 percent correct must be achieved to demonstrate satisfactory completion of each chapter, but you are encouraged to review difficult-to-grasp material until you are satisfied that you have learned it completely.

LEARNING OBJECTIVES

Academic Objectives. Upon completion of this self-study text, the student will be able to:

1 State definitions for general terminology used in parasitology.
2 Recall the scientific and common names for each parasite studied.
3 State the general geographic distribution of each parasite.
4 State the parasitic form that causes disease in humans and its body location.
5 Describe the means by which each infection occurs.
6 State the name of the disease produced and its most common symptoms and pathology.
7 State the appropriate body specimen to examine for the diagnostic stage of each parasite, and list other laboratory tests useful in its diagnosis.
8 Recognize and draw the diagnostic stage of each parasite.
9 Demonstrate graphically the life cycle of each parasite.
10 Discuss the procedures used to identify parasites (including concentration, culture, and staining techniques), as well as potential sources of error involved and quality-control procedures.
11 Identify potentially successful methods for the epidemiologic control of parasitism.
12 Given sufficient case history information, identify the most probable helminth or protozoan causing the symptoms and the body specimen of choice for study.

Practical Objectives. Upon completion of this self-study text and with appropriate experiences in the laboratory, the student will:

1 Be able to perform appropriate and satisfactory microscopic and macroscopic examination of body specimens—such as blood, urine, or feces—to detect and to identify parasites (acceptable performance is the identification of at least 80 percent of the parasites present in specimens).
2 Have mastered two fecal concentration techniques (one for sedimentation and one for flotation) as demonstrated by satisfactory performance of these techniques and correct identification of recovered parasites.
3 Be able to prepare and to stain slides of fecal material and blood satisfactorily as demonstrated by the correct diagnosis of at least 80 percent of the parasites contained therein.
4 Be able to perform a variety of other tests satisfactorily, including a fecal egg count, a blood concentration test for microfilariae, and serodiagnostic testing for various parasites.

PRE-TEST The following questions will help you evaluate your general knowledge of parasitology. Allow 20 minutes for completion of the test. The multiple-choice questions are worth **6**

points each; questions 11 and 12 are worth **20 points** each. Write your answers on separate sheets of paper.

1. Pinworm disease may be diagnosed by which procedure?
   a. Direct fecal smear
   b. Cellophane tape test
   c. Fecal concentration methods
   d. Egg-count technique

2. *Taenia solium* tapeworm infection occurs when:
   a. Undercooked beef is eaten
   b. Eggs are ingested from contaminated soil
   c. Larvae invade the skin of the feet
   d. Undercooked pork is eaten

3. The most common helminth infection in the United States is:
   a. *Necator americanus*
   b. *Ascaris lumbricoides*
   c. *Enterobius vermicularis*
   d. *Schistosoma mansoni*

4. The definitive host for *Plasmodium vivax* is a:
   a. Flea
   b. Human
   c. Mosquito
   d. Fish

5. *Clonorchis sinensis* is commonly known as the:
   a. Beef tapeworm
   b. Hookworm
   c. Chinese liver fluke
   d. Bladder worm

6. The most pathogenic ameba in humans is:
   a. *Entamoeba histolytica*
   b. *Entamoeba coli*
   c. *Giardia lamblia*
   d. *Balantidium coli*

7. Which of the following may be used to culture amebae in the laboratory?
   a. Horse serum
   b. Wheatley trichrome
   c. Loose moist soil
   d. Balamuth medium

8. Xenodiagnosis is used for which parasite?
   a. *Schistosoma mansoni*
   b. *Trypanosoma cruzi*
   c. *Loa loa*
   d. *Wuchereria bancrofti*

9. Diptera is an order of insects including which of the following?
   a. Mosquitoes
   b. Lice
   c. Fleas
   d. Bugs
   e. Ticks

10. The common name for *Necator americanus* is:
    a. Pinworm
    b. Trichina worm
    c. Hookworm
    d. Fish tapeworm

11. Match the disease in the left column with the correct causative parasite in the right column:
    a. _____ Dwarf tapeworm disease
    b. _____ Threadworm disease
    c. _____ Traveler's diarrhea
    d. _____ Liver rot
    e. _____ Whipworm disease

    1. *Giardia lamblia*
    2. *Fasciola hepatica*
    3. *Hymenolepis nana*
    4. *Trichuris trichiura*
    5. *Strongyloides stercoralis*

12. Define or explain the following terms:
    a. Vector
    b. Host
    c. Proglottid
    d. Definitive host
    e. Operculum

The answer key to all tests starts on page 167.

CLASSIFICATION OF PARASITES

I. Helminths—Metazoa; wormlike invertebrates. (Only those parasitic for humans are included in this text.) The following will be considered:
   A. Phylum Nemathelminthes
      1. Class Nematoda: roundworms (body round in cross-section)
   B. Phylum Platyhelminthes: flatworms
      1. Cestoda: tapeworms (body flattened and segmented)
      2. Class Digenea: trematodes, flukes (body flattened, leaf-shaped, and nonsegmented)
II. Protozoa*—unicellular eukaryotic microorganisms. The following will be considered:
   A. Phylum Sarcomastigophora
      1. Class Lobosea: organisms that move by means of pseudopodia
      2. Class Zoomastigophorea: organisms that move by means of flagella
   B. Phylum Ciliophora
      1. Class Kinetofragminophorea: organisms that move by means of cilia
   C. Phylum Apicomplexa
      1. Class Sporozoea: organisms with both sexual and asexual reproductive cycles; **apical complex** seen with electron microscope
III. Arthropods—hard exoskeleton, jointed appendages. Only those that are parasitic to humans and those that transmit parasitic diseases will be considered.
   A. Phylum Arthropoda
      1. Class Insecta: flies, mosquitoes, bugs, lice, fleas
      2. Class Arachnida: ticks, mites

GLOSSARY OF GENERAL TERMINOLOGY

Six glossaries of important terms appear in this text. In addition to the basic terms defined below, separate glossaries are included in the chapters on the Nematoda, Cestoda, Digenea, Protozoa, and Arthropoda.

Study and master all the words in each of the glossaries. It is recommended that the glossaries be used in conjunction with the bold-faced terms appearing in the text. A medical dictionary will also be helpful. Before taking each post-test, review the glossary included in the chapter.

accidental or incidental host. Infection of a host other than the normal host species. A parasite may or may not continue full development in an accidental host.

apical complex. Polar complex of secretory organelles in sporozoan protozoa.

carrier. A host harboring a parasite but exhibiting no clinical signs or symptoms.

commensalism. The association of two different species of organisms in which one partner is benefited and the other is neither benefited nor injured.

definitive host. The host animal in which a parasite passes its adult existence and/or sexual reproductive phase.

differential diagnosis. The clinical comparison of different diseases that exhibit similar symptoms designed to determine from which the patient is suffering.

disease. A definite morbid process having a characteristic train of symptoms.

ectoparasite. A parasite established on or in the exterior surface of a host.

endoparasite. A parasite established within the body of its host.

epidemiology. A field of science dealing with the relationships of the various factors that determine the frequency and distribution of an infectious process or disease in a community.

facultative parasite. An organism capable of living an independent or a parasitic existence; not an obligatory parasite, but potentially parasitic.

generic name (or scientific name). The name given to an organism consisting of its appropriate genus and species title.

genus (pl. genera). A taxonomic category subordinate to family (and tribe) and superior

---

*Classification derived from scheme adopted by Society of Protozoologists (from Cox, 1993).

to species, grouping those organisms that are alike in broad features but different in detail.

host. The species of animal or plant that harbors a parasite and provides some metabolic resources to the parasitic species.

in vitro. Observable in a test tube or other nonliving system.

in vivo. Within the living body.

infection. Invasion of the body by a pathogenic organism (except arthropods), with accompanying reaction of the host tissues to the presence of the parasite.

infestation. The establishment of arthropods upon or within a host (including insects, ticks, and mites).

intermediate host. The animal in which a parasite passes its larval stage or asexual reproduction phase.

Metazoa. A subkingdom of animals consisting of all multicellular animal organisms in which cells are differentiated to form tissue. Includes all animals except Protozoa.

obligatory parasite. A parasite that cannot live apart from its host.

parasitemia. The presence of parasites in the blood (e.g., malaria schizonts in red blood cells).

parasitism. The association of two different species of organisms in which the smaller species lives upon or within the other and has a metabolic dependence on the larger host species.

pathogenic. Production of tissue changes or disease.

pathogenicity. The ability to produce pathogenic changes.

reservoir host. An animal that harbors a species of parasite that is also parasitic for humans and from which a human may become infected.

serology. The study of antibody-antigen reactions in vitro, using host serum for study.

species (abbr. **spp.**). A taxonomic category subordinate to a genus. A species maintains its classification by not interbreeding with other species.

symbiosis. The association of two different species of organisms exhibiting metabolic dependence by their relationship.

vector. Any arthropod or other living carrier that transports a pathogenic microorganism from an infected to a noninfected host. A vector may transmit a disease passively (mechanical vector) or may be an essential host in the life cycle of the pathogenic organism (biologic vector).

BIBLIOGRAPHY   **General References**

American Society of Medical Technology Staff: *Clinical Diagnostic Parasitology,* ed 3. Kendall-Hunt, Dubuque, Iowa, 1992.

Benke, JM (ed): *Parasites, Immunity and Pathology: The Consequences of Parasitic Infection in Mammals.* Taylor and Francis, New York, 1990.

Binford, CH, and Connor, DH: *Pathology of Tropical and Extraordinary Diseases,* Vols 1 and 2. Armed Forces Institute of Pathology, Washington, DC, 1990.

Campbell, WC, and Rew, RS (eds): *Chemotherapy of Parasitic Diseases.* Plenum Press, New York, 1986.

Cheng, TC: *General Parasitology,* ed 2. Academic Press, New York, 1986.

Cheng, TC, et al: *Parasitic and Related Diseases: Basic Mechanisms, Manifestations and Control.* Plenum Press, New York, 1986.

Cook, GC: *Parasitic Disease in Clinical Practice.* Springer-Verlag, London, 1990.

Cox, FEG (ed): *Modern Parasitology,* ed 2. Blackwell Scientific Publication, Oxford, 1993.

Daws, B (ed): *Advances in Parasitology.* Academic Press, London and New York, volumes published annually since 1962.

Esh, GW, and Fernandez, J: *Functional Biology of Parasitism: Ecological and Evolutionary Implications.* Chapman and Hall, New York, 1993.

Faust, EC, Beaver, PC, and Jung, RC: *Animal Agents and Vectors of Human Disease,* ed 4. Lea & Febiger, Philadelphia, 1975.

Goldsmith, R, and Hayneman, D: *Tropical Medicine and Medical Parasitology.* Appleton & Lange, Norwalk, Connecticut, 1989.

Leach, RM, and Jeffery, HC: *Atlas of Medical Helminthology and Protozoology,* ed 3. Churchill, New York, 1991.

MacLeod, C (ed): *Parasitic Infections of Pregnancy and the Newborn.* Oxford University Press, New York, 1988.

Markell, EK, Vogue, M, and John, DT: *Medical Parasitology,* ed 7. WB Saunders, Philadelphia, 1992.

Schmidt, GD, and Roberts, LS: *Foundations of Parasitology,* ed 4. CV Mosby, St Louis, 1981.

Science, Vol 264, No 5167, pp 1857–1886. 24 June, 1994.

Soulsby, EJL (ed): *Immune Responses in Parasitic Infections: Immunology, Immunopathology and Immunoprophylaxis,* 4 Vols. CRC Press, Boca Raton, Florida, 1987.

Strickland, GT (ed): *Hunter's Tropical Medicine,* ed 7. WB Saunders, Philadelphia, 1991.

Sun, T: *Color Atlas and Textbook of Diagnostic Parasitology.* Igaku-Shoin, Tokyo, New York, 1988.

Symons, LE: *Pathophysiology of Parasitic Infections.* Academic Press, New York, 1989.

Taylor, AER, and Baker, JR (eds): *In Vitro Methods for Parasite Cultivation.* Academic Press, New York, 1988.

Warren, KS, and Mahmoud, AAF: *Tropical and Geographical Medicine,* ed 2. McGraw-Hill, New York, 1990.

Wyler, DJ (ed): *Modern Parasite Biology: Cellular, Immunological and Molecular Aspects.* WH Friedman, New York, 1990.

CHAPTER 2

Nematoda

LEARNING OBJECTIVES

Upon completion of this chapter and the supplementary color plates as described, the student will be able to:

1   Define terminology specific for **Nematoda**.
2   State the scientific and common names for all intestinal nematodes for which humans serve as the usual definitive host.
3   State the body specimen of choice to be used for examination to diagnose nematode infections.
4   State the geographic distribution and relative incidence of nematodes of medical importance.
5   Describe the general morphology of an adult nematode.
6   Describe the development of parasitic intestinal nematodes from egg through adult stages.
7   Differentiate the adult parasitic intestinal Nematoda.
8   Given an illustration or photograph or an actual specimen (if given adequate laboratory experience), identify the diagnostic stages of intestinal Nematoda.
9   Differentiate microfilariae found in infected human blood.
10   Discuss zoonotic nematode infections of humans and symptoms thereof.
11   Classify, differentiate, and discuss methods by which the Nematoda infect humans. Include the scientific name of any required intermediate host and the infective stage for humans.
12   Perform generic identification of parasitic infections by detecting, recognizing, and stating the scientific name of parasites present in biologic laboratory specimens (given appropriate laboratory experiences, as described in Chapter 7).

Use these learning objectives as guides for your acquisition of knowledge. Assure yourself that you have indeed acquired the information necessary to do each task described before you attempt a chapter post-test.

The class Nematoda includes both free-living species that are metabolically independent and parasitic species that have a metabolic dependence on a host species in order to continue their life cycle. As a group, the nematodes are referred to as roundworms because they are round when viewed in cross section. The different species vary in size from a few millimeters to over a meter in length. There are separate sexes, with the male being generally smaller than the female. The male frequently has a curved or coiled posterior end with **copulatory spicules** and, in some species, a **bursa**. The adult anterior end may have oral hooks, teeth, or plates in the **buccal capsule**, for the purpose of attachment, and small body surface projections, known as setae or papillae, which are thought to be sensory in nature. Body development is fairly complex. The exterior resistant surface of the adult worm is called the **cuticle**; this is underlain with several muscle layers. The internal organ systems include a complex nerve cord; a well-developed digestive system (buccal capsule, muscular esophagus, gut, and anus); and complete, tubular, coiled reproductive organs, which are proportionally very large and complex. In the male, these include testes, vas deferens, seminal vesicle, and an ejaculatory duct. The female reproductive organs include two ovaries, oviducts, uterine seminal receptacle, and vagina. The female can produce from several hundred up to millions of offspring, depending upon the species. **Fecundity** is usually proportional to the complexity of the life cycle of the parasite.

Humans are the definitive host for the roundworms of medical importance, inasmuch as they harbor the reproducing adult roundworms. The adult female nematode produces fertilized eggs, or larvae, which may be infective to a new host by one of three routes: Eggs may be immediately infective by being ingested, eggs or larvae may require a period of development to reach the infective stage, or eggs may be transmitted to a new host by an insect. Developing larvae generally go through a series of four **molts**. Most often it is the third-stage larva (the **filariform stage**) that is infective. Infection of humans with roundworms can be by ingestion of the infective stage egg or larva, by larval penetration through the skin of the host, or via transmission of larvae by the bite of an insect.

The development of a parasite to the infective stage and the manner in which humans become infected are different for each parasite species.

Of the species of nematodes parasitic for humans, about half reside as adult worms in the intestinal tract; the others are found as adults in various human tissues. The pathogenicity of intestinal nematodes may be due, in part, to migration of larvae through body tissues to the intestines, piercing of the intestinal wall, bloodsucking activities of the

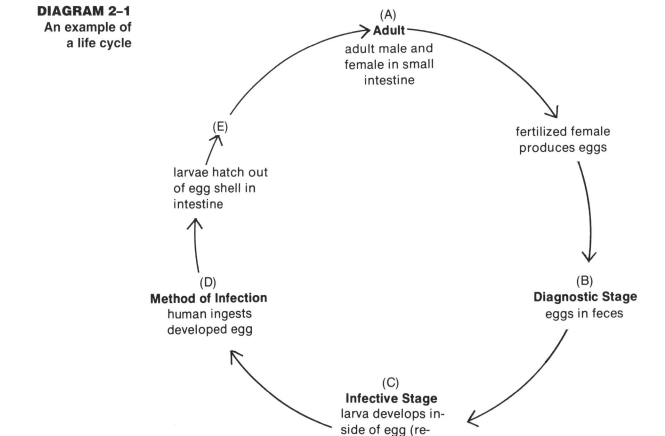

DIAGRAM 2–1
An example of a life cycle

(A)
Adult
adult male and female in small intestine

fertilized female produces eggs

(B)
Diagnostic Stage
eggs in feces

(C)
Infective Stage
larva develops inside of egg (requires 2 to 4 weeks in moist warm soil)

(D)
Method of Infection
human ingests developed egg

(E)
larvae hatch out of egg shell in intestine

worms, or allergic reactions to substances secreted by either adult worms or larval stages. This can be serious in heavy infections. Pathogenicity induced by the tissue roundworms is primarily due to immune and nonspecific host responses to the parasite secretions and excretions and to degenerating parasite material. Most infected persons have low worm burdens and modest symptoms. Migrating nematodes are usually associated with blood and/or tissue **eosinophilia**.

Diagram 2–1 is a generalized example of a **life cycle** that will show you the key points to study while learning about any parasite. Understanding the life cycle is the key to understanding how to break the cycle in nature and thereby control the transmission of parasitic diseases. Minimally, the five parts noted on the diagram of the life cycle must be known.

A. Location of the parasite stage in a human host (e.g., adults in intestinal tract).
B. The means by which parasite stages leave the human host (e.g., eggs in feces). This is usually the parasite stage that is seen and identified in the laboratory. A parasite stage that is so recognized in any biologic specimen and thus serves as a key to diagnosis is termed the **diagnostic stage**.
C. The parasite stage that is infective to humans is termed the **infective stage**. It must be noted if external development is required for the parasite to reach infectivity (e.g., eggs develop in the soil) or if a part of the life cycle is spent in another host.
D. The means by which a new human host is infected (e.g., egg is ingested).
E. Sites of development and maturation of the parasite in humans.

GLOSSARY   **Nematoda.** A class of the animal phylum Nemathelminthes—the roundworms.

buccal capsule (cavity). Oral cavity of roundworms. (In the case of hookworms, the cavity contains either cutting plates or cutting teeth.)

bursa (pl. **bursae**). Fan-shaped cartilage expansion at the posterior end of some male nematodes (e.g., hookworms).

copulatory spicules. Needlelike bodies possessed by some male nematodes; spicules lie in pouches near ejaculatory duct and may be inserted in the vagina of the female worm during copulation.

corticated. Possessing an outer, mamillated, albuminous coating, as on the eggs of *Ascaris lumbricoides*.

cutaneous larval migrans. A disease caused by the migration of larvae of *Ancylostoma* spp. (dog or cat hookworm) or other helminth under the skin of humans. Larval migration is marked by thin, red papular lines of eruption. Also termed creeping eruption.

cuticle. The surface of roundworms; a tough protective covering that is resistant to digestion.

dermatitis. Inflammation of the skin.

diagnostic stage. A developmental stage of a pathogenic organism that can be detected in human body secretions, discharges, feces, blood, or tissue by chemical means or microscopic observations as an aid in diagnosis.

diurnal. Occurring during the daytime.

edema. Unusual excess fluid in tissue, causing swelling.

elephantiasis. Overgrowth of the skin and subcutaneous tissue that is due to obstructed circulation in the lymphatic vessels; occurs in the presence of some long-term filaria infections (e.g., *Wuchereria bancrofti*).

embryonation. The development of a fertilized helminth embryo into a larva.

enteritis. Inflammation of the intestine.

eosinophilia. High levels of circulating eosinophils in the blood.

fecundity. Reproductive capacity.

filaria (pl. **filariae**). A nematode worm of the order Filariata; requires an arthropod intermediate host for transmission.

filariform larva. Infective, nonfeeding, sheathed, third-stage larva; long, slender esophagus.

gravid. Pregnant; female has developing eggs, embryos, or larvae in reproductive organs.

immunosuppression. Depressed immune response system; can accompany various diseases or be drug-induced.

incubation period. The time from initial infection until the onset of clinical symptoms of a disease.

infective stage. The stage of a parasite at which it is capable of entering the host and continuing development within the host.

intermediate host. A species of animal that serves as host for only the larval or sexually immature stages of parasite development. Required part of the life cycle of that parasite.

larva (pl. **larvae**). An immature stage in the development of a worm before it becomes a mature adult. Nematodes **molt** several times during development, and each subsequent larval stage is increasingly mature.

life cycle. Entrance into a host, growth, development, reproduction, and transmission of a parasite to a new host.

microfilaria (pl. **microfilariae**). A term used for the embryo of a filaria, usually in the blood or tissue of humans; ingested by the arthropod intermediate host.

molt. A process of replacement of the old cuticle with an inner, new one and subsequent shedding of the old, outer cuticle to allow for the growth and development of the larva; the actual shedding of the old cuticle is termed ecdysis.

occult. Hidden; not apparent.

parthenogenic. Capable of unisexual reproduction; no fertilization is required, e.g., *Strongyloides stercoralis* parasitic female.

periodicity. Recurring at a regular time period.

pica. Habit of eating dirt or other unusual substances, such as chalk or plaster. Seen most often in children or in adults with anemia.

prepatent period. The time elapsing between initial infection with the parasite and reproduction by the adult parasite.

pruritus. Intense itching.

rectal prolapse. Weakening of the rectal musculature resulting in a "falling down" of the rectum; occasionally seen in heavy whipworm infections, particularly in children.

rhabditiform larva. Noninfective, feeding, first-stage larva; has an hourglass-shaped esophagus.

tropical eosinophilia. A disease syndrome associated with high levels of blood eosinophils and an asthmalike syndrome. Caused by zoonotic filaria (or other nematode) infections in which there are usually no microfilariae detectable in peripheral blood.

visceral larval migrans. A disease in humans caused by the migration of the roundworm *Toxocara canis* or *T. cati* through the liver, lungs, or other organs. The normal host of these ascarids is the dog or cat. The disease is characterized by hypereosinophilia and hepatomegaly, and frequently by pneumonia. Migrating larvae can invade ocular spaces and cause retinal damage.

zoonosis (pl. **zoonoses**). A disease involving a parasite for which the normal host is an animal but that has accidentally infected a human.

INTESTINAL NEMATODES

In Table 2–1 you will find listed the scientific names (genus and species names) and also the common names for the intestinal roundworms of medical importance that are included in this section. On the following pages are the life cycle diagrams, disease names, some of the major pathology and symptoms caused by infection with these roundworms, distribution, and other points of diagnostic importance. (See Color Plates 1–27 and accompanying descriptions.) When you complete the study of these organisms, you should be able to write

1. The scientific name
2. The common name
3. The location of the adults in humans
4. The diagnostic stage and body specimen of choice for examination
5. The method of infection of humans
6. Other specific information pertinent to the diagnosis of each parasitic infection

	Table 2–1. INTESTINAL ROUNDWORMS	
Order	**Scientific Name (Genus and Species)**	**Common Name**
Ascaridida	*Enterobius vermicularis* (en"tur-o'bee-us/vur-mick-yoo-lair'is)	pinworm, seatworm
Tricocephalida	*Trichuris trichiura* (trick-yoo'ris/trick"ee-yoo'ruh)	whipworm
Ascaridida	*Ascaris lumbricoides* (as'kar-is/lum-bri-koy'deez)	large intestinal roundworm
Strongylida	*Necator americanus* (ne-kay'tur/ah-merr"i-kay'nus)	New World hookworm
Strongylida	*Ancylostoma duodenale* (an"si-los'tuh-muh/dew'o-de-nay'lee)	Old World hookworm
Rhabditida	*Strongyloides stercoralis* (stron"ji-loy'-deez/stur"ko-ray'lis)	threadworm
Tricocephalida	*Trichinella spiralis* (trick"i-nel'uh/spy-ray'lis)	trichina worm

Proper pronunciation of the scientific name is given beneath each name. Practice pronouncing the scientific name aloud and spelling it on paper.

In addition to the life cycle charts, Table 2–2 (page 23) will help you review the pertinent information for each parasite, including the **epidemiology** and the major disease manifestations caused by these parasites. The second section of this chapter covers the tissue nematodes in the same manner as the intestinal nematodes, and the third section discusses zoonotic diseases. Be sure to also study the corresponding pictures and descriptive key found in the color atlas at the front of the book while learning the text material. All other chapters of this book follow the same format.

When you feel you have mastered these materials (as outlined in the learning objectives), you are ready to take the post-test on the section. The directions for each test are included on the test pages, and the answer key begins on page 167.

DIAGRAM 2–2
Enterobius vermicularis
(pinworm, seatworm)

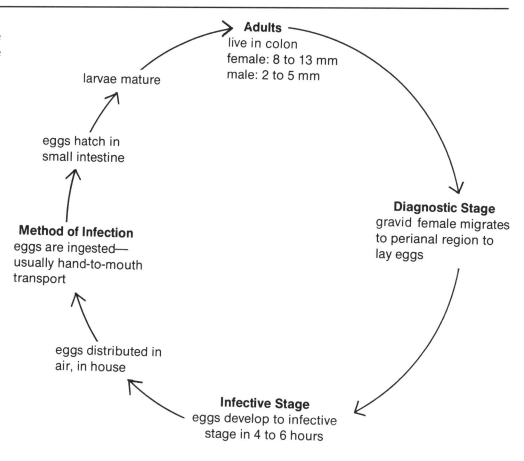

Adults
live in colon
female: 8 to 13 mm
male: 2 to 5 mm

larvae mature

eggs hatch in
small intestine

Method of Infection
eggs are ingested—
usually hand-to-mouth
transport

Diagnostic Stage
gravid female migrates
to perianal region to
lay eggs

eggs distributed in
air, in house

Infective Stage
eggs develop to infective
stage in 4 to 6 hours

METHOD OF DIAGNOSIS   Recover eggs or yellowish-white adult from perianal region with a cellophane tape preparation taken early in the morning when the patient first wakes. (See Chapter 7, page 132.)

DIAGNOSTIC STAGE

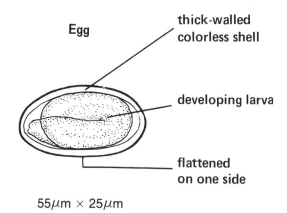

Egg

thick-walled
colorless shell

developing larva

flattened
on one side

55μm × 25μm

DISEASE NAMES   Enterobiasis, pinworm infection

MAJOR PATHOLOGY AND SYMPTOMS

1. Many cases are asymptomatic. Infrequently causes severe clinical problems.
2. Rarely causes serious lesions; usually limited to minute ulcers and mild inflammation of intestine. Abdominal pain in about half of reported symptoms.
3. Other symptoms are associated with the migration of the **gravid** female out from the anus to lay her eggs on the perianal region at night.

a. Cardinal feature is hypersensitivity reaction causing severe perianal itching; eggs get on hands from scratching; pruritus ani is pathognomonic.
b. Mild nausea or vomiting.
c. Loss of sleep, irritability.
d. Slight irritation to intestinal mucosa.
e. Vulval irritation in girls from migrating worms entering vagina.

TREATMENT Mebendazole or pyrantel pamoate. Warm tap water enemas. May need to treat the whole family because eggs are easily spread in the environment.

DISTRIBUTION Worldwide, but more prevalent in temperate climates. Higher incidence in whites than in blacks. Most common helminth infection in the United States. It is a group infection, especially common among children.

OF NOTE
1. Humans are the only known host. Infection is generally self-limiting.
2. Each female produces up to 15,000 eggs. Most eggs become infective within 4 hours of release and remain infective for only a few days. Cleaning eggs from the environment and treating all persons in the household are important in order to break the life cycle.
3. Eggs are rarely found in fecal samples because release is external to the intestine. Adult females can be recovered occasionally on cellophane tape preparation used to find eggs on perianal area.
4. Hatched larvae on perianal area may migrate back into rectum and large intestine and develop to adults (retroinfection), or autoreinfection (ingestion of eggs) can occur.

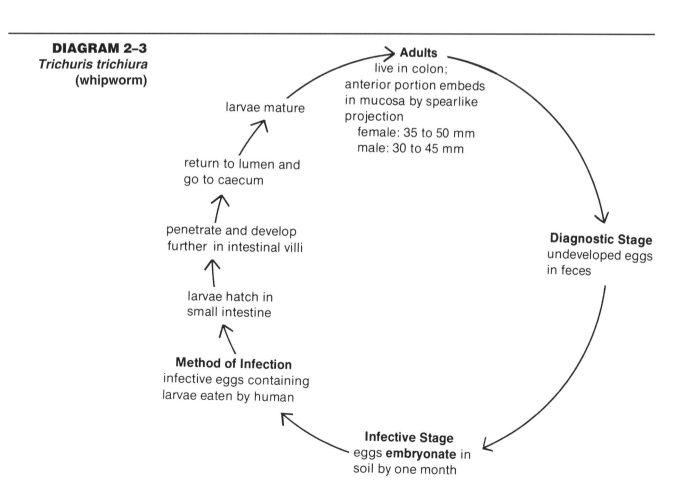

DIAGRAM 2–3
Trichuris trichiura
(whipworm)

larvae mature

Adults
live in colon;
anterior portion embeds
in mucosa by spearlike
projection
 female: 35 to 50 mm
 male: 30 to 45 mm

return to lumen and
go to caecum

penetrate and develop
further in intestinal villi

larvae hatch in
small intestine

Method of Infection
infective eggs containing
larvae eaten by human

Diagnostic Stage
undeveloped eggs
in feces

Infective Stage
eggs **embryonate** in
soil by one month

METHOD OF DIAGNOSIS   Recovery and identification of characteristic eggs in feces

DIAGNOSTIC STAGE

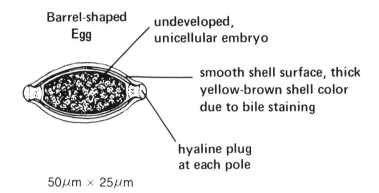

Barrel-shaped Egg

undeveloped, unicellular embryo

smooth shell surface, thick yellow-brown shell color due to bile staining

hyaline plug at each pole

$50\mu m \times 25\mu m$

DISEASE NAMES   Trichuriasis, whipworm infection

MAJOR PATHOLOGY AND SYMPTOMS
1. Slight infection—asymptomatic. No treatment required.
2. Heavy infection (500 to 5000 worms) simulates ulcerative colitis in children and inflammatory bowel disease in adults. Histology reveals eosinophil infiltrations but no decrease in goblet cells. Surface of colon matted with worms; patient will have
   a. Bloody or mucoid diarrhea.
   b. Weight loss and weakness.
   c. Abdominal pain and tenderness; colitis may be seriously debilitating.
   d. Increased peristalsis and rectal prolapse, especially in children.
3. Chronic infections in children can stunt growth.
4. Stool loose with mucus (and obvious blood) in heavy infection.

TREATMENT   Mebendazole

DISTRIBUTION   Prevalent in warm countries and areas of poor sanitation. In the United States, prevalent in the warm, humid climate of the South. Third most common intestinal helminth. More common among children and institutionalized mentally retarded.

OF NOTE
1. Commonly, double infections occur with *Ascaris* because of the similar method of human infection, that is, ingestion of eggs from soil. **Pica** common in children.
2. Drug treatment may cause production of distorted eggs, which will have bizarre shapes when seen in a fecal specimen.
3. **Zoonosis** infection can occur with pig or dog whipworm.

DIAGRAM 2–4
Ascaris lumbricoides
(large intestinal roundworm)

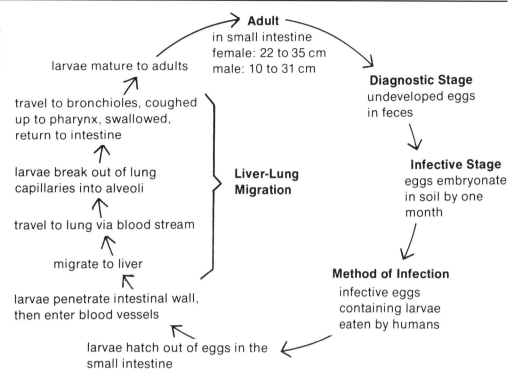

> **Adult**
> in small intestine
> female: 22 to 35 cm
> male: 10 to 31 cm

larvae mature to adults

travel to bronchioles, coughed
up to pharynx, swallowed,
return to intestine

larvae break out of lung
capillaries into alveoli

travel to lung via blood stream

migrate to liver

larvae penetrate intestinal wall,
then enter blood vessels

**Liver-Lung
Migration**

Diagnostic Stage
undeveloped eggs
in feces

Infective Stage
eggs embryonate
in soil by one
month

Method of Infection
infective eggs
containing larvae
eaten by humans

larvae hatch out of eggs in the
small intestine

**METHOD OF
DIAGNOSIS** Recovery and identification of fertile (corticated or not) or infertile eggs in feces. Sedimentation concentration test recommended instead of flotation. Enzyme-linked immunosorbent assay (ELISA) serologic test available.

**DIAGNOSTIC
STAGE**

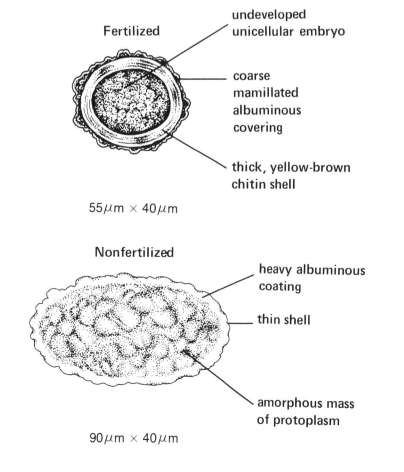

Fertilized

undeveloped
unicellular embryo

coarse
mamillated
albuminous
covering

thick, yellow-brown
chitin shell

55μm $\times$ 40μm

Nonfertilized

heavy albuminous
coating

thin shell

amorphous mass
of protoplasm

90μm $\times$ 40μm

DISEASE NAMES   Ascariasis, roundworm infection

MAJOR PATHOLOGY AND SYMPTOMS

1. Tissue phase: pneumonia, cough, low-grade fever, and 30 to 50 percent eosinophilia (Löffler's syndrome) due to migration of larvae through the lungs (1 to 2 weeks after ingestion of eggs). Allergic asthmatic reaction may occur with reinfection.
2. Intestinal phase: intestinal or appendix obstruction by adults in heavy infections.
   a. Vomiting and abdominal pain due to adult migration.
   b. Protein malnutrition in children with heavy infections and poor diets.
   c. Some patients are asymptomatic.
3. Complications from obstruction due to tangling of the large worms or from migration of adults to other sites, such as appendix, bile duct, or liver (detectable by x ray).
4. Adults may exit by nose, mouth, or anus. Large, creamy white, with tapered anterior; male has curved tail.

TREATMENT

1. Mebendazole or pyrantel pamoate.
2. Piperazine citrate.
3. Levamisole.
4. Corticosteroid treatment helps symptoms of severe pulmonary phase.
5. Nasogastric suction and drug treatment, or surgery, for intestinal obstruction by adults.

DISTRIBUTION   Prevalent in warm countries and areas of poor sanitation. Coexists with *T. trichiura* in the United States; found predominantly in the Appalachian Mountains and adjacent regions to the east, south, and west. The eggs of these two species require the same soil conditions for development to the infective state, and infection for both is by ingestion of infective eggs.

OF NOTE

1. *Ascaris* is the largest adult intestinal nematode.
2. Adults are active migrators provoked by fever, certain drugs, and anesthesia, and may tangle and block intestine or migrate through intestine or appendix and out of the mouth or anus. Mortality is due mainly to intestinal complications.
3. *Ascaris* is the second most common intestinal helminth infection in the United States and the most common infection on a worldwide basis.
4. The adult female lays up to 250,000 eggs per day.
5. Eggs may remain infective in soil or water for years; resistant to chemicals.

DIAGRAM 2–5
Necator americanus
(New World
hookworm) and
*Ancylostoma
duodenale* (Old World
hookworm)

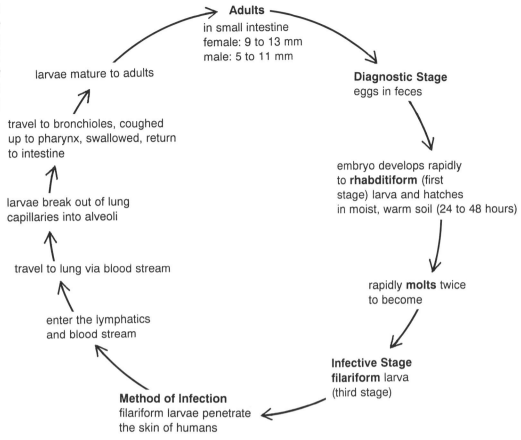

Adults
in small intestine
female: 9 to 13 mm
male: 5 to 11 mm

larvae mature to adults

travel to bronchioles, coughed
up to pharynx, swallowed, return
to intestine

larvae break out of lung
capillaries into alveoli

travel to lung via blood stream

enter the lymphatics
and blood stream

Method of Infection
filariform larvae penetrate
the skin of humans

**Infective Stage
filariform** larva
(third stage)

rapidly **molts** twice
to become

embryo develops rapidly
to **rhabditiform** (first
stage) larva and hatches
in moist, warm soil (24 to 48 hours)

Diagnostic Stage
eggs in feces

**METHOD OF
DIAGNOSIS** Recovery and identification of hookworm eggs in fresh or preserved feces. Cannot differentiate species by egg appearance.

**DIAGNOSTIC
STAGE**

(*Note:* **Eggs of these species
are almost identical.**)

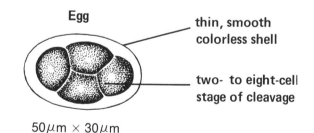

Egg

thin, smooth
colorless shell

two- to eight-cell
stage of cleavage

50μm × 30μm

DISEASE NAME Hookworm disease

**MAJOR
PATHOLOGY AND
SYMPTOMS**
1. After repeated infection, severe allergic itching at site of skin penetration by infective larvae, known as "ground itch." Penetration stings and erythematous papule forms.
2. Migration of larvae through lungs: intra-alveolar hemorrhage and mild pneumonia with cough, wheezing, sore throat, bloody sputum, and headache in heavy infections.
3. Intestinal phase of infection:
   a. Acute (heavy worm burden—showing more than 5000 eggs per gram [EPG] of feces): **enteritis**, epigastric distress in 20 to 50 percent, anorexia, diarrhea, pain, microcytic hypochromic iron-deficiency anemia with accompanying weakness, signs of hypoproteinemia, edema, and loss of strength due to blood loss caused by adult worms.

    b. Chronic (light worm burden—showing fewer than 500 EPG): the usual form of this infection; slight anemia, weakness, or weight loss; nonspecific mild gastrointestinal symptoms (may be subclinical).

    c. Symptoms secondary to the iron-deficiency anemia. Hyperplasia of bone marrow and spleen.

    d. High eosinophilia.

TREATMENT   Mebendazole or pyrantel pamoate; iron replacement therapy. Thiabendazole ointment for **cutaneous larval migrans**.

DISTRIBUTION   *Necator americanus*—North and South America; Asia; including China and India; and Africa.

    Ancylostoma duodenale—Europe; South America; Asia, including China; Africa; and the Caribbean.

    Other species in the Far East.

    Common in agrarian areas with poor sanitation.

    Almost one-quarter of world population assumed to be infected.

OF NOTE

1. Moist, warm regions and bare-skin contact with sandy soil are optimal conditions for contracting heavy infections in areas of poor sanitation. Often found in same soil conditions as *Ascaris* and *Trichuris.*

2. Delayed fecal examination can result in egg hatching and larval development; therefore, *Strongyloides* larvae must be differentiated from hookworm larvae (see color plates). Hookworm rhabditiform larvae have a long buccal capsule; *Strongyloides* rhabditiform larvae have a short buccal capsule.

3. Adults are voracious bloodsuckers; heavy infection can result in 100 mL of blood loss per day; therefore, provide dietary and iron therapy support along with drug treatment as necessary.

4. Other animal species of hookworm larvae can migrate through the human dermis after penetration, causing allergic reaction in the migration tracks (cutaneous larval migrans).

5. Differentiate adults by buccal capsule and bursa (see color plates).

6. *Ancylostoma* filariform larvae can also infect orally and possibly by transmammary or transplacental passage.

7. Pica contributes to infection and is a common symptom.

DIAGRAM 2–6
Strongyloides stercoralis (threadworm)

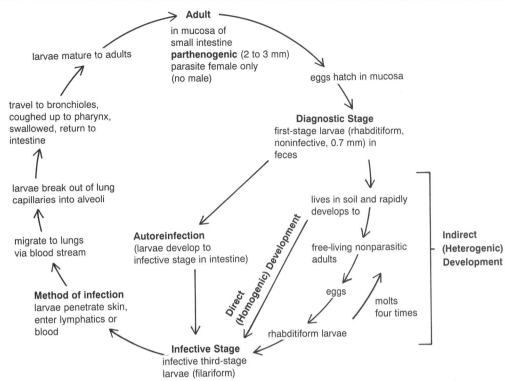

Adult
in mucosa of small intestine **parthenogenic** (2 to 3 mm) parasite female only (no male)

larvae mature to adults

travel to bronchioles, coughed up to pharynx, swallowed, return to intestine

larvae break out of lung capillaries into alveoli

migrate to lungs via blood stream

Method of infection
larvae penetrate skin, enter lymphatics or blood

eggs hatch in mucosa

Diagnostic Stage
first-stage larvae (rhabditiform, noninfective, 0.7 mm) in feces

Autoreinfection
(larvae develop to infective stage in intestine)

Direct (Homogenic) Development

lives in soil and rapidly develops to

free-living nonparasitic adults

eggs

molts four times

rhabditiform larvae

Indirect (Heterogenic) Development

Infective Stage
infective third-stage larvae (filariform)

METHOD OF DIAGNOSIS

Recovery and identification of **rhabditiform** larvae in feces. Present in low numbers. Also, presence of hookwormlike eggs or larvae in duodenal drainage fluid or from Enterotest capsule is diagnostic. (Larvae must be differentiated from hookworm larvae when found in feces; see color plate key.) Serology: ELISA. Larvae may be in sputum in disseminated strongyloidiasis. In severe cases, x ray shows loss of mucosal pattern rigidity and tubular narrowing.

DIAGNOSTIC STAGE

Rhabditiform larva
(*Note:* Egg resembles hookworm egg.)

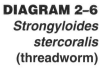

short buccal cavity

hourglass-shaped esophagus

genital primordium

anus

275μm × 16μm

DISEASE NAMES

Strongyloidiasis, threadworm infection

MAJOR PATHOLOGY AND SYMPTOMS

1. Major clinical features are abdominal pain, diarrhea, and urticaria, with eosinophilia.
2. Skin: recurring allergic, raised, itchy, red wheals from larval penetration.
3. Migration of larvae: primary symptoms are in lungs; bronchial verminous pneumonia.
4. Intestine: abdominal pain, diarrhea and constipation, vomiting, weight loss, variable anemia, eosinophilia, protein-losing enteropathy. Frequently asymptomatic in light

infection; gross lesions usually absent; bowel is edematous and congested in heavy infection.

5. Has caused sudden deterioration and death in immunocompromised persons because of heavy autoinfection and larval migration throughout body (hyperinfection), with bacterial infection secondary to larval spread and intestinal leakage.

TREATMENT Thiabendazole (not always successful); albendazole, ivermectin.

DISTRIBUTION Warm areas, tropics, and subtropics worldwide; similar to hookworm.

OF NOTE

1. Parasitic female is **parthenogenic**; therefore, can have multiplication and autoinfection in the same host.
2. Internal infection can continue for years because of maintenance of autoinfection.
3. Strongyloidiasis is difficult to treat.
4. Often defective T-lymphocyte function.
5. *Strongyloides* larvae do not float in saturated salt solutions; sedimentation concentration preferred.

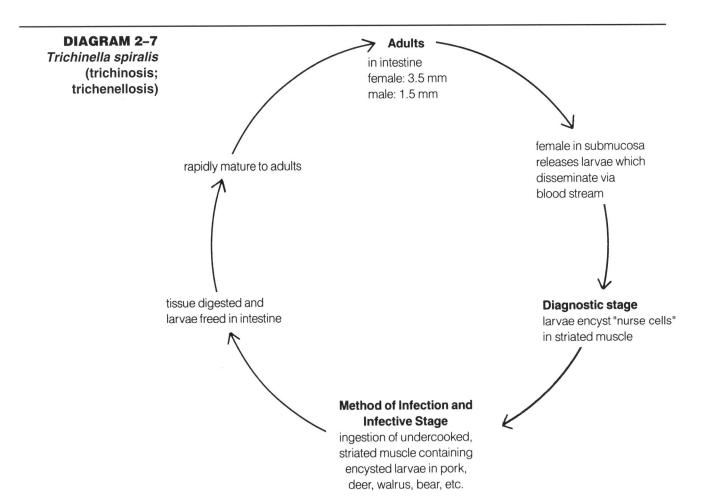

DIAGRAM 2–7
Trichinella spiralis
**(trichinosis;
trichenellosis)**

Adults
in intestine
female: 3.5 mm
male: 1.5 mm

female in submucosa
releases larvae which
disseminate via
blood stream

rapidly mature to adults

tissue digested and
larvae freed in intestine

Diagnostic stage
larvae encyst "nurse cells"
in striated muscle

**Method of Infection and
Infective Stage**
ingestion of undercooked,
striated muscle containing
encysted larvae in pork,
deer, walrus, bear, etc.

**METHOD OF
DIAGNOSIS** Identification of encysted larvae in biopsied muscle: serologic testing (ELISA) 3 to 4 weeks following infection. A history of eating undercooked pork or bear; fever, muscle pain, bilateral periorbital edema, and rising eosinophilia warrants presumptive diagnosis.

DIAGNOSTIC STAGE

Larva encysted in a muscle cell (called the "nurse cell")

(Note: **Granuloma forms around nurse cell and becomes calcified over time.**)

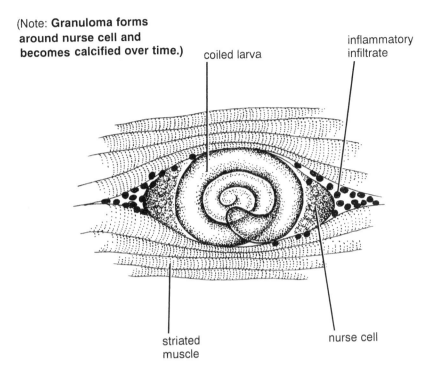

coiled larva

inflammatory infiltrate

striated muscle

nurse cell

DISEASE NAMES Trichinosis, trichinellosis

MAJOR PATHOLOGY AND SYMPTOMS

1. Intestinal phase: small intestine edema and inflammation; nausea, vomiting, abdominal pain, diarrhea, headache, and fever (first week after infection).
2. Migration phase: high fever (104°F), blurred vision, edema of the face and eyes, cough, pleural pains, eosinophilia (15% to 40%) lasting one month with heavy infection; death can occur during this phase in 4th to 8th week following infection.
3. Muscular phase: acute local inflammation with edema and pain of the musculature. Other symptoms variable, depending on the location and number of larvae present. Larvae encyst in skeletal muscles of limbs, diaphragm, and face but invade other muscles as well. Weakness and fatigue.
4. Focal lesions: periorbital edema, splinter hemorrhages of fingernails, retinal hemorrhages, rash.

DISTRIBUTION Worldwide among meat-eating populations, rare in tropics. Prevalence in the United States about 4 percent based on autopsy studies; about 100 cases recognized and reported per year in the United States.

TREATMENT

1. Non-life-threatening infection (self-limiting): rest, analgesics, and antipyretics.
2. Life-threatening: prednisone. Thiabendazole (caution—effectiveness not proven, may have side effects).

OF NOTE

1. Zoonosis: Carnivorous mammals are primary hosts. Found in most species.
2. Multiple cases often related to one source of infected meat.

DIAGRAM 2–8
*Dracunculus
medinensis*
(guinea worm)

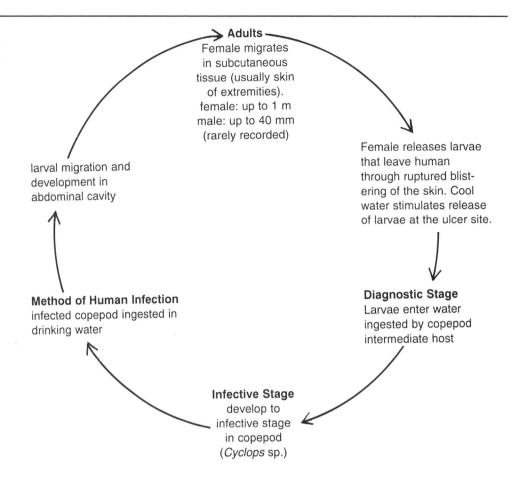

Adults
Female migrates
in subcutaneous
tissue (usually skin
of extremities).
female: up to 1 m
male: up to 40 mm
(rarely recorded)

Female releases larvae
that leave human
through ruptured blist-
ering of the skin. Cool
water stimulates release
of larvae at the ulcer site.

larval migration and
development in
abdominal cavity

Method of Human Infection
infected copepod ingested in
drinking water

Diagnostic Stage
Larvae enter water
ingested by copepod
intermediate host

Infective Stage
develop to
infective stage
in copepod
(*Cyclops* sp.)

METHOD OF DIAGNOSIS   Visual observation of painful skin blister, emerging worm; induced release of larvae from skin ulcer when cold water is applied.

MAJOR PATHOLOGY AND SYMPTOMS
1. Allergic reaction during migration.
2. Papule developing into a blister that ruptures, usually on feet or legs.
3. Secondary bacterial infections or reaction to aberrant migration of larvae or adults may cause disability or death.

TREATMENT   Remove adult from skin (slow withdrawal from blister or remove surgically). Aspirin for pain. Prevent secondary infection.

DISTRIBUTION   Middle East, India, Pakistan, and Africa

OF NOTE
1. Largest adult nematode.
2. No effective immunity to reinfection.
3. WHO is sponsoring attempt at global eradication through promotion of drinking water filtration (tee shirts or gauze can be used) to strain copepods, plus education campaign to keep people out of water when adult worms protrude from body.

Table 2–2. IMPORTANT INTESTINAL NEMATODE INFECTIONS

Scientific and Common Name	Epidemiology	Disease-Producing Form and Its Location in Host	How Infection Occurs	Major Disease Manifestations, Diagnostic Stage, and Specimen of Choice
Enterobius vermicularis (pinworm)	Worldwide	Adult worms in colon; eggs on perianal region	Infective eggs are discharged by the gravid female on perianal skin; eggs are transferred from hand to mouth	Perianal itching caused by local irritation from scratching Diagnosis: eggs found by cellophane test (page 132)
Trichuris trichiura (whipworm)	Worldwide, especially in moist, warm climate	Adult worms in colon	Ingestion of eggs containing mature larvae from infected soil or food	Light infection—asymptomatic Heavy infection—enteritis, diarrhea, rectal prolapse Diagnosis: eggs in feces
Ascaris lumbricoides (large intestinal roundworm)	Worldwide, especially in moist, warm climate	Larval migration through liver and lungs Adult worms in small intestine	Ingestion of eggs containing mature larvae from infected soil or food	Light infection—asymptomatic Heavy infection—pneumonia from larval migration Diarrhea and bowel or appendix obstruction Diagnosis: eggs or adults in feces
Trichinella spiralis (trichina worm)	Worldwide	Adults in small intestine Larval migration; larvae encyst in striated muscle	Ingestion of encysted larva in undercooked meat (pork or bear)	Gastric distress, fever, eye edema, acute muscle pain, eosinophilia Diagnosis: encysted larvae in muscle biopsy; serology
Necator americanus (New World hookworm)	U.S., West Africa, Asia, and South Pacific	Larval migration; ground itch Adults in small intestine	Eggs shed in feces, mature in soil, larvae hatch and mature Infective (filariform) larvae penetrate host skin, especially feet	Repeated infection results in larval dermatitis with later pulmonary symptoms Microcytic hypochromic anemia from chronic blood loss if heavy infection and poor diet Diagnosis: eggs in feces
Ancylostoma duodenale (Old World hookworm)	Europe, Brazil, Mediterranean area, and Asia	As above (for *Necator americanus*)	As above	As above
Strongyloides stercoralis (threadworm)	Worldwide, warm areas	Larval migration; pulmonary signs Adults in small intestine	Immature (rhabditiform) larvae are shed in feces, develop in soil Infective (filariform) larvae penetrate host skin, especially feet Autoreinfection by maturing larvae in intestine *continued on next page*	Repeated infection results in larval dermatitis with later pulmonary symptoms Heavy infections—abdominal pain, vomiting, and diarrhea Moderate eosinophilia *continued on next page*

Table 2-2. IMPORTANT INTESTINAL NEMATODE INFECTIONS Continued

Scientific and Common Name	Epidemiology	Disease-Producing Form and Its Location in Host	How Infection Occurs	Major Disease Manifestations, Diagnostic Stage, and Specimen of Choice
			Soil dwelling, nonparasitic adults may produce additional infective-stage larvae	Immunosuppressed host may suffer severe symptoms or death from heavy worm burdens inasmuch as autoinfection may occur Diagnosis: rhabditiform larvae in feces
Dracunculus medinensis (Guinea worm)	Africa, Asia, South America No periodicity *Cyclops* (crustacean)	Adults live in subcutaneous tissues; females migrate (larvae released from skin ulcer)	Ingestion of water containing crustaceans infected with larvae	Systemic allergic symptoms and local ulcer formation Diagnosis: adult in skin ulcer, larvae released into water

Proceed now to the front of the book to study Color Plates 1 to 27 and accompanying discussions.

FILARIAE: TISSUE NEMATODES

Table 2–3 gives the scientific and common names for the members of the superfamily Filarioidea (the tissue roundworms) to be discussed in this section.

GENERAL LIFE CYCLE

Adult filariae live in various human tissue locations. In general, fertilized adult female filariae living in the tissues produce living embryos (**microfilariae**), which migrate into lymphatics, blood, or skin. All these parasites require an arthropod **intermediate host** for transmission of infection. If the arthropod ingests microfilariae while taking a blood meal, they molt twice inside the arthropod intermediate host and become the infective stage filariform larvae. These larvae are released from the insect's proboscis and enter a new human definitive host when the arthropod next feeds on blood. The entering larvae migrate to the appropriate tissue site and develop to become adults. Maturation can take up to a year.

Table 2-3. FILARIAE

Scientific Name	Common Name
Wuchereria bancrofti (wooch-ur-eer'ee-uh/ban-krof'tye)	Bancroft's filaria
Brugia malayi (broog'ee-uh/may-lay eye)	Malayan filaria
Loa loa lo'uh/lo'uh)	eyeworm
Onchocerca volvulus (onk'o-sur'kuh/vol'vew-lus)	blinding filaria

In some species, the microfilariae are more prevalent in peripheral blood at specific times of the day or evening (i.e., they exhibit **periodicity**). These times appear to coincide with the usual feeding pattern of the arthropod intermediate host species. Nocturnal or **diurnal** periodicity is noted in Table 2–4.

At least three other species of filariae are common parasites of humans. *Mansonella perstans*, found in Africa and Central and South America, and *Mansonella ozzardi*, found in Central and South America, apparently do not induce pathology but do produce microfilariae in the blood. *Mansonella streptocerca*, found in tropical Africa, is also non-pathogenic but produces microfilariae that are found in the skin like *Onchocerca volvulus*. Microfilariae in blood or tissue must, therefore, be speciated, and these diagnostic stages are illustrated to aid in differential diagnosis of filariasis.

Information listed on the following pages is keyed by number according to genus and species: **1** = *Wuchereria bancrofti*; **2** = *Brugia malayi*; **3** = *Loa loa*; **4** = *Onchocerca volvulus*.

Table 2–4. IMPORTANT FILARIAL INFECTIONS

Scientific and Common Name	Epidemiology, Periodicity, and Intermediate Host	Disease-Producing Form and Its Location in Host	How Infection Occurs	Major Disease Manifestations, Diagnostic Stage, and Specimen of Choice
Wuchereria bancrofti (Bancroft's filaria)	Tropics Nocturnal periodicity *Culex, Aedes*, and *Anopheles* mosquitoes	Adults live in the lymphatics (microfilariae in blood)	Filariform larvae enter through bite wound into the blood when the mosquito bites a human to take a blood meal	Invades lymphatics and causes granulomatous lesions, chills, fever, eosinophilia, and eventual elephantiasis Diagnosis: microfilariae in blood; serology
Brugia malayi (Malayan filaria)	Far East Nocturnal periodicity *Anopheles* and *Mansonia* mosquitoes	As above	As above	As above
Loa loa (eyeworm)	Africa Diurnal periodicity *Chrysops* fly	Adults migrate throughout the subcutaneous tissues (microfilariae in blood)	As above, except the vector is a bloodsucking fly	Chronic and benign disease Diagnosis: microfilariae in blood; serology; Calabar swelling (a transient, subcutaneous swelling)
Onchocerca volvulus (blinding filaria)	Central America and Africa No periodicity *Simulium* (blackfly)	Adults live in fibrotic nodules (microfilariae migrate subcutaneously)	As above, except the vector is a bloodsucking fly	Chronic and nonfatal Allergy to microfilariae causes local symptoms—may cause blindness Diagnosis: adults in excised nodules; microfilariae in tissue scraping of nodule

DIAGRAM 2–9
Filariae

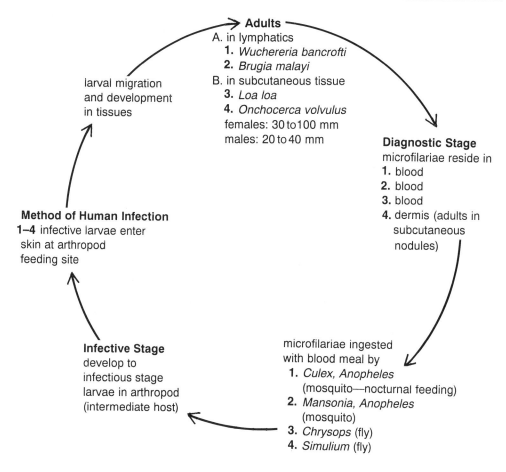

Adults
A. in lymphatics
  1. *Wuchereria bancrofti*
  2. *Brugia malayi*
B. in subcutaneous tissue
  3. *Loa loa*
  4. *Onchocerca volvulus*
  females: 30 to 100 mm
  males: 20 to 40 mm

larval migration
and development
in tissues

Diagnostic Stage
microfilariae reside in
1. blood
2. blood
3. blood
4. dermis (adults in
  subcutaneous
  nodules)

Method of Human Infection
1–4 infective larvae enter
skin at arthropod
feeding site

microfilariae ingested
with blood meal by
  1. *Culex, Anopheles*
    (mosquito—nocturnal feeding)
  2. *Mansonia, Anopheles*
    (mosquito)
  3. *Chrysops* (fly)
  4. *Simulium* (fly)

Infective Stage
develop to
infectious stage
larvae in arthropod
(intermediate host)

METHOD OF DIAGNOSIS

A. **1–3.** (Numbers refer to organisms in Diagram 2–9.) Microfilariae (200 to 300 μm) in stained blood smear (see page 134). Also, can centrifuge blood sample and lyse red blood cells to concentrate microfilariae in the specimen before staining. (See page 135, Knott technique.)
4. Microfilariae in tissue scraping of nodule.
B. Serology (lacks specificity).

Differentiation of Microfilariae as Seen in a Stained Blood Smear

Examine for the presence or absence of a sheath (a thin, translucent eggshell remnant covering the body of the microfilaria and extending past the head and tail).

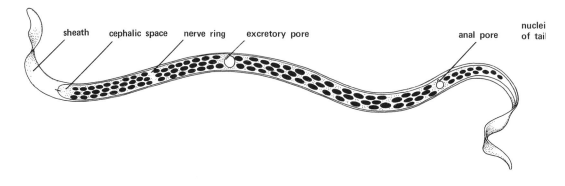

sheath   cephalic space   nerve ring   excretory pore   anal pore   nuclei of tail

Examine tail area of microfilaria for presence or absence of cells that exhibit a characteristic array of stained nuclei.

A. No nuclei in tailtip

(A1) *Wuchereria bancrofti*
sheath present

(A2) *Mansonella ozzardi* **(nonpathogen)**
no sheath

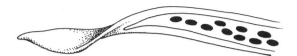
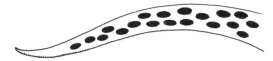

Tail of microfilaria of *Onchocerca volvulus* as seen in a tissue scraping from the nodular mass containing the adult filaria or from a skin snip (no sheath; nuclei not terminal, tail straight).

Tail of *Mansonella streptocerca* microfilaria is bent like a fishhook. These microfilariae are not found in blood smears, only in tissue scrapings.

(A3) *Onchocerca Volvulus*

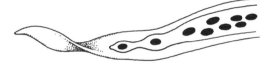

B. Nuclei in tail

(B1) *Loa loa*
**continuous row of posterior nuclei;
sheath present**

(B2) *Brugia malayi*
**nuclei not continuous, two at
tip of tail; sheath present**

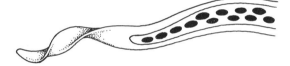
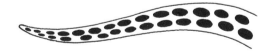

(B3) *Mansonella perstans* **(nonpathogen)**
nuclei in tip of tail; no sheath

DISEASE NAME Filariasis

1. Elephantiasis, Bancroft's filariasis
2. Malayan filariasis
3. Eyeworm
4. Blinding filaria; river blindness

MAJOR PATHOLOGY AND SYMPTOMS Diagnosis is difficult because symptoms are broad-spectrum. Depends on identification of microfilariae.

1–2. Early acute phase causes fever and lymphangitis; after years of repeated exposure chronic elephantiasis develops because of obstruction of lymphatics, lymph stasis, and lymphedematous changes. Adults in lymphatics sequentially induce dilation, inflammation, and, after death of the adult worm, surrounding granulomatous thickening of lymphatic walls, and, finally, obstruction. Malayan filariasis is more often asymptomatic. In endemic areas, "filaria fevers" are seen, with recurrent acute lymphangitis and adenolymphangitis without microfilariae. Also seen is tropical eosin-

ophilia syndrome or Weingarten's syndrome (which resembles asthma) with high eosinophilia and no microfilariae.
3. Localized subcutaneous edema (Calabar swellings), particularly around eye, because of microfilariae migration and death in capillaries (more serious in visitors to endemic area). Living adults cause no inflammation; dying adults induce granulomatous reaction. Proteinuria. Endomyocardial fibrosis (EMF).
4. Fibrotic nodules encapsulating adults (onchocercomas). Progressively severe allergic onchodermatitis (pigmented rash); blindness occurs from the presence of microfilariae in all ocular structures (very prevalent in Africa and in Central America [on coffee plantations]).

TREATMENT
1. Diethylcarbamazine; ivermectin kills microfilariae
2. Diethylcarbamazine
3. Diethylcarbamazine (also prophylactic)
4. Ivermectin

DISTRIBUTION
1. Spotty worldwide, tropical and subtropical
2. East and Southeast Asia
3. Rainforest belt in Africa and Sudan
4. Central America and equatorial Africa

OF NOTE
1. Mosquito's resistance to insecticides and increasing coastal-dwelling human populations are increasing the incidence of exposure.
2. Eosinophilic lung (tropical eosinophilia), an asthmalike syndrome, may be caused by **occult** filariasis or zoonotic infection.
3. Onchocerciasis is the major cause of blindness in Africa; control is difficult because *Simulium* breeds in running water.
4. Filarial infection can induce an "immunosuppressed state" in the host that prevents a reaction to the parasite, but immune-mediated inflammatory responses or immunologic hyperreactive immunopathology (elephantiasis response) can still occur.

Proceed now to the front of the book to study Color Plates 28 to 33 and accompanying descriptions.

ZOONOSES   Zoonoses are infections in humans by parasites that usually live in animals. Table 2–5 lists the scientific names of the parasites, their geographic locations, their normal animal hosts, and the disease and symptoms produced in humans following accidental infection. These parasites do not normally develop full life cycles in humans.

Table 2–5. IMPORTANT ZOONOTIC INFECTIONS

Scientific and Common Name	Geographic Location	Normal Animal Host	Disease	Symptoms in Humans	Method of Infection of Humans
Ancylostoma braziliense *Ancylostoma caninum* (dog hookworms)	Southern U.S., Central and South America, Africa, Asia, Northern Hemisphere	Dog and cat Dog	Cutaneous larval migrans (CLM); Creeping eruption	Allergic response to the migration of larvae under the skin Red, itchy tracts, usually on legs	Penetration of the skin by filariform larvae
Angiostrongylus cantonensis (rat lungworm)	China, Hawaii, and tropical islands	Rat	Eosinophilic meningoencephalitis	Eosinophilia and symptoms of meningitis; turbid spinal fluid contains many white blood cells, including increased eosinophils (looks like coconut juice)	Ingestion of infected snail or prawn (intermediate host)
Angiostrongylus costaricensis	Central America	Rat		Adult worms lay eggs in mesenteric arteries near cecum; cause granulomas and abdominal inflammation	Eating unwashed vegetables contaminated with mucous secretions from infected slug (intermediate host)
Anisakis spp. (roundworm of marine mammals and fish)	Japan, Netherlands	Herring, other fish	Eosinophilic granuloma in stomach or small intestine	Abdominal pain and an eosinophilic granuloma around the migrating larvae of *Anisakis* in the intestinal wall	Ingesting raw fish containing the larval stage
Capillaria philippinensis	Far East	Fish		Malabsorption syndrome; extreme and persistent diarrhea; death from cardiac failure or secondary infection. Adults multiply in human intestine and cause blockage	Ingestion of infected raw fish
Dirofilaria spp. (filariae of canines)	Various species worldwide	Dog, raccoon, fox	Tropical eosinophilia, eosinophilic lung	High eosinophilia, chronic cough, pulmonary infiltrates, high levels of IgE Microfilariae are rarely present in peripheral blood	Bite of mosquito vector carrying infective filaria larvae
Gnathostoma spp.	Far East	Dog, feline		Acute visceral larval migrans syndrome; then intermittent chronic subcutaneous swellings. Invades nervous system in Southeast Asia	Ingestion of larva from raw, infected fish, or application of infected snake poultice to open lesion; larvae migrate into lesion
Gongylonema pulchrum	Worldwide	Pig		Migrating worm in facial subcutaneous tissue	Accidental ingestion of infected roach or dung beetle
Thelazia spp.	Worldwide	Various mammals		Habitation of conjunctival sac or lacrimal duct by adult; severe irritation of eye	Contact with infected fly or roach

Table continued on next page

Table 2–5. IMPORTANT ZOONOTIC INFECTIONS Continued

Scientific and Common Name	Geographic Location	Normal Animal Host	Disease	Symptoms in Humans	Method of Infection of Humans
Toxocara canis; *T. cati* (large intestinal roundworms of dogs or cats)	Worldwide	Dog, cat	Visceral larval migrans (VLM) or systemic toxocariasis Ocular toxocariasis	Eosinophilia, elevated isohemagglutinins, hepatomegaly, pulmonary inflammation with cough and fever; often history of seizures; alternative to VLM is possible encystment of the larvae in the eye (ocular larval migrans), which mimics a malignant tumor (retinoblastoma) All symptoms due to migration of larvae in the tissues of humans	Ingestion of infective-stage larvae in developed eggs from soil History of pica in children and exposure to puppies

You have now completed the chapter covering the Nematoda. After reviewing this material and the related color plates with descriptions, using the learning objectives to direct your studies, proceed to the first post-test. Allow 45 minutes to complete the test. Write your answers on a separate piece of paper. The answers are given in the back of the book. If you answer fewer than 80 percent of the questions correctly, review all the appropriate material and retake the test. Follow this procedure for all chapter post-tests. Follow up with review of areas that need strengthening.

BIBLIOGRAPHY   **Intestinal Nematodes**

Banwell, JG, and Schad, GA: Hookworm. *Clinics in Gastroenterology* 7:129–156, 1978.

Behnke, JM: Evasion of immunity by nematode parasites causing chronic infections. Adv Parasitol 26:2–71, 1987.

Bundy, DAP, and Cooper, ES: Trichuris and trichuriasis in humans. Adv Parasitol 28:108–173, 1989.

Crompton, DW, et al (eds): *Ascariasis and Its Public Health Significance.* Taylor & Francis, Philadelphia, 1985.

Crompton, DWT: Hookworm disease: Current status and new directions. Parasitology Today 5:1–2, 1989.

Cruz, T, Reboucas, G, and Rocha, H: Fatal strongyloidiasis in patients receiving corticosteroids. N Engl J Med 275:1093, 1966.

Giles, HM, and Ball, PAJ: Hookworm infection. In Ruitenberg, EJ and Macinnis, AJ (eds): *Human Parasitic Diseases*, Vol 4. Elsevier, New York, 1991.

Gillas, HM: Selective primary health care: Strategies for control of disease in the developing world. XVII. Hookworm infection and anemia. Review of Infectious Diseases 7:111–118, 1985.

Gould, SE: *Trichinosis in Man and Animals.* Charles C Thomas, Springfield, IL, 1970.

Grove, SS, and Elsdon-Dew, R: Internal auto-infection with *Strongyloides stercoralis.* South African Journal of Laboratory and Clinical Medicine 4:55, 1958.

Layrisse, M, Aparcedo, L, Martinez-Torres, C, et al: Blood loss due to infection with *Trichuris trichiura.* Am J Trop Med Hyg 16:613, 1967.

O'Brien, W: Intestinal malabsorption in acute infection with *Strongyloides stercoralis.* Trans R Soc Trop Med Hyg 69:69, 1975.

Roche, M, and Layrisse, M: The nature and causes of "hookworm anemia." Am J Trop Med Hyg 15:1031, 1966.

Schad, G, and Warren, K (eds): *Hookworm Disease: Current Status and New Directions.* Taylor and Francis, Philadelphia, 1990.

Sodeman, TM, and Dock, N: Laboratory diagnosis of parasitic and fungal diseases of the central nervous system. Ann Clin Lab Sci 6:47, 1976.

Thune, O: Creeping eruption of larval migrans. Int J Dermatol 11:231, 1972.

Filariae

Beverley-Burton, M, and Crichton, VF: Identification of guinea-worm species. Trans R Soc Trop Med Hyg 67:152, 1973.

Choyce, DP: Epidemiology and natural history of onchocerciasis. Isr J Med Sci 8:1143, 1972.

Choyce, DP: Onchocerciasis: Ophthalmic aspects. Trans R Soc Trop Med Hyg 60:720, 1966.

CIBA Foundation Staff: *Filariasis*, No. 127. Wiley, New York, 1987.

Coolidge, C, et al: Zoonotic *Brugia* filariasis in New England. Ann Intern Med 90:341, 1979.

Danaraj, TJ, Pacheco, G, Shanmugaratnam, K, et al: The etiology and pathology of eosinophilic lung (tropical eosinophilia). Am J Trop Med Hyg 15:183, 1966.

Nelson, GS: *Onchocerciasis*. In Dawes, B (ed): *Advances in Parasitology*, Vol 8. Academic Press, New York, 1970.

Nelson, GS: Current concepts in parasitology: Filariasis. N Engl J Med 300:1136, 1979.

Nutman, TB, et al: *Loa loa* infection in temporary residents in endemic region: Recognition of a hyperresponsive syndrome with characteristic clinical manifestations. J Infect Dis 154:10–18, 1986.

Ottesen, EA: Immunopathology of lymphatic filariasis in man. Springer Semin Immunopathol 2:373, 1980.

Ottesen, EA: Immunological aspects of lymphatic filariasis and onchocerciasis in humans. Trans R Soc Trop Med Hyg 78(suppl): 9–18, 1984.

Otteson, RE: Description, mechanisms and control of post-treatment reactions in human filiariasis. Ciba Found Symp 127:265–283, 1987.

Price, EW: The mechanism of lymphatic obstruction in endemic elephantiasis of the lower legs. Trans R Soc Trop Med Hyg 69:177, 1975.

Sasa, M: *Human Filariasis*. University Park Press, Baltimore, 1976.

Woodruff, AW: Toxocariasis. Br Med J 3:663, 1970.

World Health Organization: Lymphatic pathology and immunopathology in filiariasis: Report of the twelfth meeting of the Scientific Working Group on Filariasis. TDR.FILSWG12 (12)/85.3, 1985.

Zoonoses

Alicata, JE, and Jindrak, K: *Angiostrongylosis in the Pacific and Southeast Asia*. Charles C Thomas, Springfield, IL, 1970.

Beaver, PC, and Orihel, TC: Human infection with the filariae of animals in the United States. Am J Trop Med Hyg 14:1010, 1965.

CRC Handbook Series in Zoonoses, Section C: *Parasitic Zoonoses*, Vols 1–3. CRC Press, Boca Raton, FL, 1982.

Danz, V, Cabrera, BD, and Canias, B, Jr: Human intestinal capillariasis, 1. Clinical features. Acta Medica Philippina 4:72, 1967.

Glickman, LP, et al: Evaluation of serodiagnostic tests for visceral larval migrans. Am J Trop Med Hyg 27:492, 1978.

Little, MD, and Most, H: Anisakid larva from the throat of a woman in New York. Am J Trop Med Hyg 22:609, 1973.

Loría-Cortez, R, and Lobo-Sanahija, JF: Clinical abdominal angiostrongylosis—A study of 116 children with intestinal eosinophilic granuloma caused by *A. costaricensis*. Am J Trop Med Hyg 29:538, 1980.

Markell, EK: Pseudohookworm infection—Trichostrongyliasis. Treatment with thiabendazole. N Engl J Med 278:831–832, 1968.

Meyers, BJ: The nematodes that cause anasakiasis. Journal of Milk and Food Technology 38:774, 1975.

Morera, P, and Cespedes, R: *Angiostrongylus costaricensis* n. sp. (Nematoda: Metastrongyloidea): A new lungworm occurring in man in Costa Rica. Rev Biol Trop 18:173, 1971.

Polnar, GO, Jr, and Jansson, HB: *Diseases of Nematodes* (2 vols). CRC Press, Boca Raton, FL, 1988.

Schlotthauer, JC, Harrison, EG, Jr, and Thompson, JH: Dirofilariasis—An emerging zoonosis? Arch Environ Health 19:887, 1969.

World Health Organization: *Parasitic Zoonoses.* WHO Technical Report No. 637, Geneva, WHO, 1979.

POST-TEST

1. Draw the life cycle of *Ascaris lumbricoides* in diagram form. Indicate the diagnostic and infective stages. **(10 points)**

2. The following was identified by the night technician. **(15 points)**

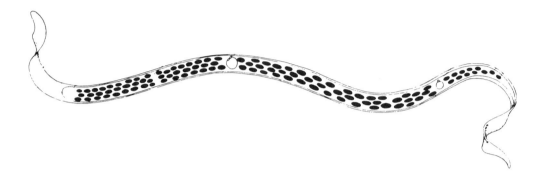

   a. What is the scientific name of the parasite?
   b. What is the intermediate host?
   c. In what body specimen was this organism identified, and what laboratory technique was helpful in finding the organism?

3. Briefly define each of the following: **(25 points)**
   a. Cutaneous larval migrans
   b. Diurnal
   c. Diagnostic stage
   d. Infective stage
   e. Prepatent stage

4. Which set of the following nematodes can cause a pneumonialike syndrome in a person exposed to heavy infection with any of the three parasites? **(15 points)**
   a. *Ascaris lumbricoides, Trichuris trichiura,* or *Onchocerca volvulus*
   b. *Enterobius vermicularis, Dracunculus medinensis,* or *Trichuris trichiura*
   c. *Strongyloides stercoralis, Wuchereria bancrofti,* or *Angiostrongylus costaricensis*
   d. *Necator americanus, Ascaris lumbricoides,* or *Strongyloides stercoralis*

5. A patient presents with vague abdominal pains and a microcytic hypochromic anemia. A possible causative parasite is: **(5 points)**
   a. *Enterobius vermicularis*
   b. *Ancylostoma duodenale*
   c. *Brugia malayi*
   d. *Trichinella spiralis*

6. An immunosupressed patient is susceptible to autoreinfection with which one of the following nematodes? **(5 points)**
   a. *Strongyloides stercoralis*
   b. *Trichinella spiralis*
   c. *Ascaris lumbricoides*
   d. *Trichuris trichiura*

7. Infection with *Enterobius vermicularis* is best diagnosed by which one of the following? **(5 points)**
   a. Examination of feces for eggs and adults

    b. Serology tests

    c. Perianal itching exhibited by patient

    d. Examination of a cellophane tape preparation for eggs and adults

8. Human infection with *Loa loa* is best diagnosed by which of the following? **(5 points)**

    a. Examination of an infected *Anopheles* mosquito

    b. Examination of blood smears

    c. Examination of feces

    d. Examination of a skin scraping

9. A child who plays in dirt contaminated with human and pet feces is susceptible to which of the following set of parasites? **(15 points)**

    a. *Ascaris lumbricoides, Trichuris trichiura, Trichinella spiralis, Wuchereria bancrofti*

    b. *Loa loa, Capillaria philippinensis, Enterobius vermicularis, Trichinella spiralis*

    c. *Strongyloides stercoralis, Toxocara canis, Ascaris lumbricoides, Nector americanus*

    d. *Ancylostoma braziliense, Trichuris trichiura, Trichinella spiralis, Necator americanus*

CHAPTER 3

Cestoda

LEARNING OBJECTIVES

Upon completion of this chapter and its supplementary color plates as described, the student will be able to:

1 State the general characteristics of phylum Platyhelminthes.
2 Compare and contrast the phylum Nemathelminthes with Platyhelminthes, using morphologic criteria.
3 Define terminology specifically related to the **Cestoda**.
4 State the scientific and common names of cestodes that parasitize humans.
5 State the methods of diagnosis used to identify cestode infections.
6 Describe the general morphology of an adult cestode.
7 Describe graphically the general life cycle of a cestode.
8 Differentiate adult Cestoda using morphologic criteria.
9 Differentiate larval stages of Cestoda using morphologic criteria and/or the required intermediate host.
10 Differentiate the diagnostic stages of the Cestoda.
11 Discuss the epidemiology and medical importance of cestode zoonoses.
12 Given illustrations or photographs (or actual specimens if you have had laboratory experience), identify diagnostic stages of Cestoda and the body specimen of choice to be used for examination for each.
13 Identify the stage in the life cycle of each cestode (including the zoonoses) that can parasitize humans.

The Platyhelminthes, as a phylum, are known as the flatworms; these are dorsoventrally flattened and have solid bodies with no body cavity. The internal organs are embedded in tissue called the parenchyma. There are no respiratory or blood-vascular systems. The life cycles of these organisms are generally indirect; that is, at least one intermediate host is required to support larval development.

The two classes of the phylum Platyhelminthes that contain human parasites are the Cestoda (the tapeworms) and the Digenea (the flukes). The Digenea are covered in Chapter 4. Platyhelminths are all **hermaphroditic** with an important exception: the blood flukes.

The external surface (termed the **tegument**) of both tapeworms and flukes is highly absorptive and even releases digestive enzymes at its surface from microtriches (specialized microvilli). The flukes have a rudimentary alimentary tract; some nutrients are taken in by mouth and some are absorbed through the tegument. The cestodes, by contrast, must absorb all nutrients through the tegument because this class of parasites has no mouth or digestive tract.

Members of the class **Cestoda** are commonly called tapeworms, inasmuch as they are long and ribbonlike and are flattened in cross-section. The adult may range from a few millimeters to 20 meters in length, depending on the species. The adult cestode lives in the intestinal tract of the vertebrate definitive host, while the larval stage inhabits tissues of the intermediate host.

The anterior end of the worm (termed **scolex**) is modified for attachment to the intestinal wall of the definitive host. The scolex is usually equipped with four cup-shaped suckers, and some species also have a crown of hooks on the scolex to aid in attachment. A scolex is less than 2 mm long, even though the whole tapeworm can be 20 m in body length. These worms have no mouth, digestive tract, or vascular system, and all nutrients are absorbed through the outer surface of the body. Waste products are released through the tegument as well. The entire body of an adult tapeworm is termed the strobila. The body of the tapeworm consists of segments known as **proglottids**. Segments form by budding from the posterior end of the scolex, an area of germinal tissue for new segment production. Older, mature segments are at the terminal end of the strobila.

Each tapeworm is hermaphroditic. Every mature proglottid of the body contains both male and female reproductive organs. The sex organs in each proglottid mature gradually so that the proglottids at the terminus of the tapeworm contain fully developed reproductive organs and the uterus is filled with fertilized eggs. (The shape of the gravid uterus is distinctive for each species.) These posterior segments are termed gravid pro-glottids and can be found singly or in short chains as they break off and are expelled in feces. The embryo seen in tapeworm eggs (termed the **onchosphere** or **hexacanth embryo**) bears six tiny hooklets that facilitate entry of the embryo into the intestinal mucosa of the intermediate host after hatching from the eggshell.

In Table 3–1 are listed the scientific names (genus and species) and the common names for the cestodes of medical importance. Use the pronunciation guide and repeat each name to yourself several times. On the following pages are shown the life-cycle diagrams of these tapeworms, and Table 3–2, page 43, reviews the pertinent information on tapeworms. Proceed to the post-test when you have learned the vocabulary and the introductory material and have mastered life cycles, Color Plates 34–52, and review table.

Table 3–1. CESTODA

Order	Scientific Name	Common Name
Cyclophyllidea	*Hymenolepis nana* (high"men-ol'e-pis/nay'nuh)	dwarf tapeworm
Cyclophyllidea	*Taenia saginata* (tee'nee-uh/sadj-i-nay'tuh)	beef tapeworm
Cyclophillidea	*Taenia solium* (tee'nee-uh/so-lee'um)	pork tapeworm
Cyclophillidea	*Echinococcus granulosus* (eh-kigh"no-kock'us/gran-yoo-lo'sus)	dog tapeworm, hydatid tapeworm
Pseudophyllidea	*Diphyllobothrium latum* (dye-fil"o-both-ree-um/lay'tum)	broad fish tapeworm

GLOSSARY **Cestoda.** A class within the phylum Platyhelminthes, which includes the tapeworms. These helminths have elongated, ribbonlike, segmented bodies.

anaphylaxis (anaphylactic shock). An exaggerated histamine-release reaction by the host's body to foreign protein, allergen, or other substances; may be fatal.

anorexia. Loss of appetite.

brood capsule. A structure within the daughter cyst in *Echinococcus granulosus* in which many scolices grow. Each scolex could develop into an adult tapeworm in the definitive host.

coracidium. A ciliated hexacanth embryo; *Diphyllobothrium latum* eggs develop to this stage and hatch then in fresh water.

cysticercoid. The larval stage of some tapeworms (e.g., *Hymenolepis nana*); a small, bladderlike structure containing little or no fluid in which the scolex is enclosed.

cysticercus. A thin-walled, fluid-filled bladderlike cyst that encloses a scolex. Also termed a bladder worm, some larvae develop in this form (e.g., *Taenia* spp.).

embryophore. The shell of *Taenia* and other tapeworm eggs as these are seen in feces.

hermaphroditic. Having both male and female reproductive organs within the same individual. All tapeworms have both sets of reproductive organs in each segment of the adult.

hexacanth embryo. A tapeworm larva having six hooklets (see **onchosphere**).

hydatid cyst. A vesicular structure formed by *E. granulosus* larvae in the intermediate host; contains fluid, brood capsules, and also daughter cysts in which the scolices of potential tapeworms are formed.

hydatid sand. Granular material consisting of free scolices, hooklets, daughter cysts, and amorphous material. Found in the fluid of older cysts of *E. granulosus.*

onchosphere. The motile, first-stage larva of certain cestodes armed with six hooklets (also termed hexacanth embryo).

operculum. The lid or caplike cover on certain platyhelminth eggs (e.g., *Diphyllobothrium latum*).

plerocercoid. The larval stage in the development of *D. latum* that develops after the procercoid stage is ingested by a freshwater fish. This form has an immature scolex and is infective if eaten by humans.

procercoid. The larval stage that develops from the coracidium of *D. latum.* It develops in the body of a freshwater crustacean.

proglottid. One of the segments of a tapeworm. Each proglottid contains male and female reproductive organs when mature.

racemose. Clusters with branching, nodular terminations resembling a bunch of grapes. Used in reference to larval cysticercosis caused by the migration and development of *T. solium* larvae in the brain tissue of humans. An aberrant form.

rostellum. The fleshy, anterior protuberance of the scolex of some tapeworms (species-specific); may bear a circular row (or rows) of hooks; may be retractable.

scolex (pl. scolices). Anterior end of a tapeworm; attaches to the wall of the intestine of a host by means of suckers and sometimes hooks.

sparganosis. Plerocercoid in human tissue from accidental infection with procercoid.

tegument (integument). The absorptive body surface of platyhelminths.

transport host. Vector; often a bloodsucking insect.

viscera (sing. viscus). Any of the large organs in the interior of any of the three great body cavities of vertebrates.

DIAGRAM 3–1
Hymenolepis nana
(dwarf tapeworm)

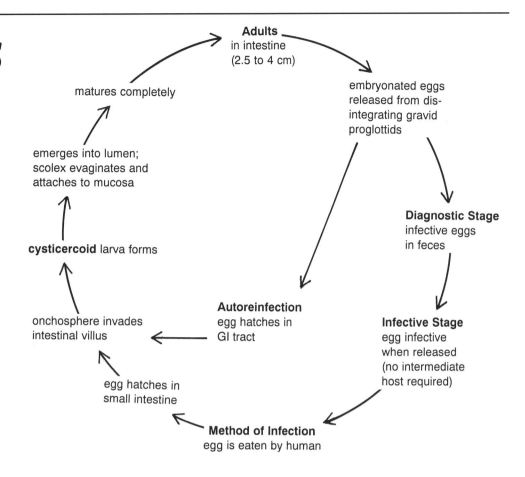

Adults
in intestine
(2.5 to 4 cm)

matures completely

embryonated eggs
released from dis-
integrating gravid
proglottids

emerges into lumen;
scolex evaginates and
attaches to mucosa

Diagnostic Stage
infective eggs
in feces

cysticercoid larva forms

Autoreinfection
egg hatches in
GI tract

Infective Stage
egg infective
when released
(no intermediate
host required)

onchosphere invades
intestinal villus

egg hatches in
small intestine

Method of Infection
egg is eaten by human

**METHOD OF
DIAGNOSIS**   Recovery and identification of eggs in feces.

**DIAGNOSTIC
STAGE**

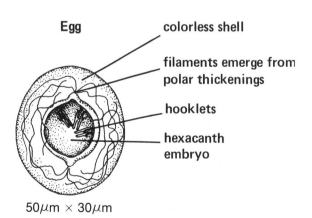

Egg
colorless shell
filaments emerge from
polar thickenings
hooklets
hexacanth
embryo

$50\mu m \times 30\mu m$

DISEASE NAME   Dwarf tapeworm infection

**MAJOR
PATHOLOGY AND
SYMPTOMS**
1. Light infection—asymptomatic.
2. Heavy infection—intestinal enteritis; abdominal pain, diarrhea, headache, dizziness, anorexia.
3. Multiple infections are common.

TREATMENT
1. Praziquantel
2. Niclosamide

DISTRIBUTION
Worldwide, tropics and subtropics, especially in children and in institutionalized persons living in close quarters. Most common human tapeworm in the United States, with greater prevalence in the Southeast, which has an estimated infection rate of 3 percent.

OF NOTE
1. The dwarf tapeworm requires no intermediate host but is also common in the house mouse, and fleas and beetles can serve as **transport hosts**. **Cysticercoid** larvae can develop in the body cavity of these insects and are infective to either humans or rodents if accidentally ingested.
2. Eggs in feces from infected mice and rats are a common source of human infection.

DIAGRAM 3–2
Taenia saginata
(beef tapeworm)
and *Taenia solium*
(pork tapeworm)

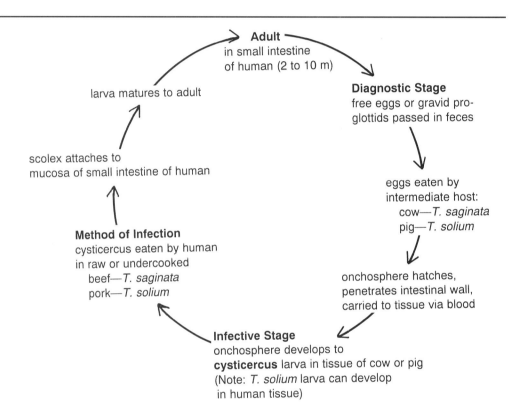

METHOD OF DIAGNOSIS
Recovery of egg or gravid proglottid (or scolex after drug treatment) in feces. For specific proglottid and scolex identification: *T. saginata* has 15 to 30 lateral uterine branches in the gravid proglottid (can be seen clearly after dye injection into the uterine pore) and a scolex with only four suckers; *T. solium* has a gravid proglottid with 7 to 12 lateral uterine branches, and the scolex has four suckers with a central crown of hooks. *T. solium* is called the ''armed'' tapeworm because of the crown of hooks by which the scolex attaches to the intestinal wall. (See Color Plate 40.) The eggs of these two species are identical.

Immunologic methods for cysticercosis: ELISA; indirect hemagglutination.

DIAGNOSTIC STAGE   Intact gravid proglottids may be found and must be differentiated. (See Color Plates 42 and 43.) Radiographic, computed tomography (CT), or magnetic resonance imaging (MRI) demonstration of *T. solium* cysticercus in tissue with signs and symptoms.

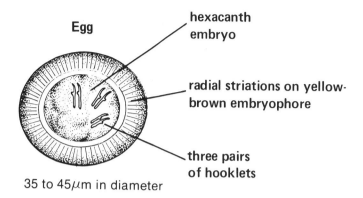

Egg

hexacanth embryo

radial striations on yellow-brown embryophore

three pairs of hooklets

35 to 45μm in diameter

DISEASE NAMES   *T. saginata*: taeniasis, beef tapeworm infection
T. solium: taeniasis, pork tapeworm infection; cysticercosis (larval infection)

MAJOR PATHOLOGY AND SYMPTOMS
1. Most infected people are asymptomatic. Abdominal pain, diarrhea, and weight loss can occur. Moderate eosinophilia.
2. Humans can serve as an intermediate host for *Taenia solium*. If eggs of *T. solium* are accidentally ingested or if eggs are released from a proglottid in the intestinal tract, the eggs can hatch in the intestine, and the larvae will migrate to form cysticercus bladders in any organ or nervous tissue (cysticercosis; neurocysticercosis [NCC] if in the central nervous system). This migration can be fatal if the **racemose** form develops in the brain. Arachnoidosis in 50 percent of active NCC cases, obstructive hydrocephalus in 25 percent. Epilepsy, headache, papilledema, vomiting.

TREATMENT   For adult tapeworm: niclosamide
For cysticercosis: praziquantel; anticonvulsants for seizures, corticosteroids for NCC symptoms; surgery

DISTRIBUTION   *T. saginata*—cosmopolitan in countries in which beef is eaten raw or insufficiently cooked. Found in southwestern United States.
T. solium—cosmopolitan when pork is eaten raw or undercooked. Rare in the United States.

OF NOTE
1. Humans are the only known definitive host for these taenias.
2. The adult worms live for many years, and usually only one worm is present in the intestine.
3. Human cysticercosis is common in Mexico and Central America.
4. Some 60 percent of patients with cysticercosis have larvae in the brain.

DIAGRAM 3–3
Diphyllobothrium latum **(broadfish tapeworm)**

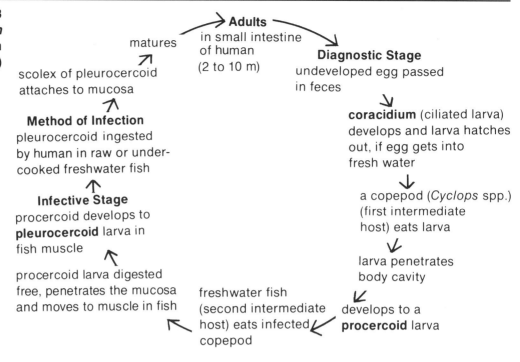

matures

> **Adults**
in small intestine
of human
(2 to 10 m)

scolex of pleurocercoid
attaches to mucosa

Diagnostic Stage
undeveloped egg passed
in feces

Method of Infection
pleurocercoid ingested
by human in raw or under-
cooked freshwater fish

coracidium (ciliated larva)
develops and larva hatches
out, if egg gets into
fresh water

Infective Stage
procercoid develops to
pleurocercoid larva in
fish muscle

a copepod (*Cyclops* spp.)
(first intermediate
host) eats larva

procercoid larva digested
free, penetrates the mucosa
and moves to muscle in fish

larva penetrates
body cavity

freshwater fish
(second intermediate
host) eats infected
copepod

develops to a
procercoid larva

METHOD OF DIAGNOSIS
Recovery of eggs in feces. Evacuated proglottids and scolices are also diagnostic in feces but are rarely naturally evacuated intact.

DIAGNOSTIC STAGE

Egg

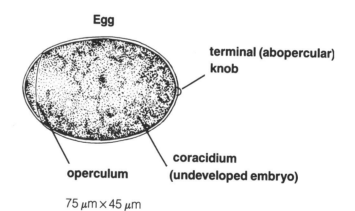

terminal (abopercular)
knob

operculum

coracidium
(undeveloped embryo)

75 μm × 45 μm

DISEASE NAMES
Diphyllobothriasis, Dibothriocephalus anemia, fish tapeworm infection, broad fish tapeworm infection.

MAJOR PATHOLOGY AND SYMPTOMS
1. Intestinal obstruction (adult can grow to 20 m) and abdominal pain. Most infected persons exhibit vague digestive symptoms.
2. Weight loss and weakness.
3. Anemia (macrocytic type) and eventual nervous system disturbances due to a B_{12} deficiency caused by the tapeworm's utilization of up to 100 percent dietary B_{12} in about 1 percent of infected persons; usually restricted to persons of Scandinavian descent.

TREATMENT
Niclosamide or praziquantel

DISTRIBUTION Temperate regions, in which freshwater fish are a common part of the diet or raw fish are eaten (the Great Lakes region of the United States, Alaska, Chile, Argentina, Central Africa, and parts of Asia). In Europe, estimates of infection include 20 percent of the Finnish people and up to 100 percent of residents of the Baltic region.

OF NOTE
1. Usually only one adult is present.
2. A variety of fish-eating mammals can serve as definitive hosts, in addition to humans.
3. The procercoid may be passed up the food chain in a dormant condition through small to larger game fish (e.g., Northern or walleyed pike).
4. A human can harbor a tissue plerocercoid if a procercoid in a copepod is ingested (see sparganosis, page 43).
5. Feces must be screened after drug treatment to ensure passage of the scolex so that no new proglottids will be formed.

DIAGRAM 3–4
Echinococcus granulosus (hydatid tapeworm)

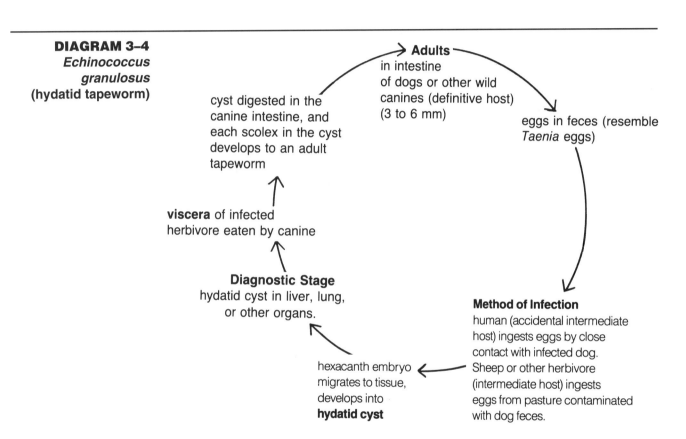

METHOD OF DIAGNOSIS
1. Serologic tests. Indirect hemagglutination (IHA), ELISA.
2. Presence of scolices, **brood capsules**, **hydatid sand**, or daughter cysts in the hydatid cyst fluid as detected by biopsy (not recommended because leakage of cyst fluid can cause **anaphylaxis**).
3. X ray, ultrasound scan, or CT detection of cyst mass in organ, especially if calcified.

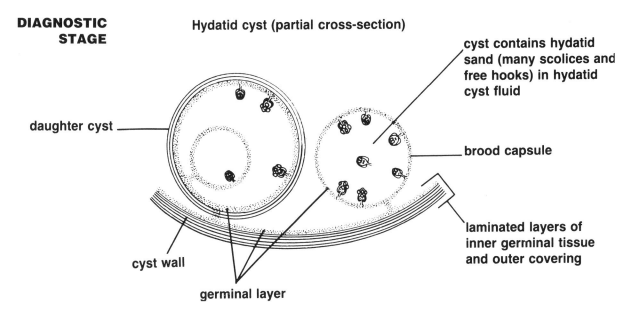

DIAGNOSTIC STAGE

Hydatid cyst (partial cross-section)

cyst contains hydatid sand (many scolices and free hooks) in hydatid cyst fluid

daughter cyst

brood capsule

laminated layers of inner germinal tissue and outer covering

cyst wall

germinal layer

DISEASE NAMES Echinococcosis, hydatid cyst, hydatid disease, hydatidosis

MAJOR PATHOLOGY AND SYMPTOMS

1. Vary according to location and size of cyst. Expanding cyst causes pressure, necrosis of surrounding tissues.
   a. In liver (most common site)—no symptoms until cyst gets large (nearly a year after ingestion of egg); can cause jaundice or portal hypertension.
   b. In lung—no symptoms until cyst becomes large; coughing, shortness of breath, chest pain.
   c. Other sites—symptoms related to enlarging cyst.
2. Cyst growth or rupture can result in death.
3. Anaphylactic shock if cyst ruptures (may occur during biopsy procedure).
4. Eosinophilia, urticaria, bronchospasm.

TREATMENT

1. Surgery
2. Mebendazole, albendazole, or praziquantel

DISTRIBUTION Cosmopolitan; human infections primarily in sheep-raising areas in which domestic dogs are used in herding.

OF NOTE

1. Hydatid disease in the United States is reported mainly in the Southwest (chiefly among the Navaho), Utah, and Alaska, and also in Canada.
2. *Echinococcus* cysts produce daughter cysts and brood capsules, all lined with germinal tissue that buds off many protoscolices, each of which will form the scolex of an adult if ingested by a canine.
3. *E. multilocularis*, which forms alveolar cysts, is rarer in humans but is intensely pathogenic and generally fatal without treatment.
4. Hydatid cyst in bone has abnormal, disseminated development in the marrow.
5. Slow-leaking cyst causes allergic sensitization. Cyst rupture (occurring naturally or during surgery) can cause anaphylaxis or spread germinal tissue to other sites in which new cysts then develop.

Table 3–2. CESTODA INFECTIONS

(A) Human Infections with Cestoda

Scientific and Common Name	Epidemiology	Disease-Producing Form and Its Location in Host	How Human Infection Occurs	Major Disease Manifestations, Diagnostic Stage, and Specimen of Choice
Hymenolepis nana (dwarf tapeworm)	Worldwide (common in southeastern United States)	Adults live in small intestine	Egg ingested by human in contaminated food or water or hand to mouth; autoreinfection is common.	Light infections—asymptomatic; heavy worm burdens cause abdominal pain, diarrhea, headaches, dizziness. Diagnosis: eggs in feces
Taenia saginata (beef tapeworm)	Cosmopolitan in beef-eating countries	Adult lives in small intestine	*Cysticercus bovis* larva eaten by human in undercooked beef	Most people are asymptomatic. Can experience abdominal pain, diarrhea, weight loss. Diagnosis: eggs or proglottid in feces
Taenia solium (pork tapeworm)	Worldwide (rare in the United States)	Adult lives in small intestine	*Cysticercus cellulosae* larva eaten by human in undercooked pork	Same as *T. saginata*
Diphyllobothrium latum (broadfish tapeworm)	Temperate areas where freshwater fish is eaten undercooked or raw	Adult lives in small intestine	Plerocercoid larva ingested by humans in freshwater fish	Can cause intestinal obstruction and macrocytic anemia due to B_{12} deficiency; abdominal pain and weight loss

(B) Accidental Zoonotic Human Infections with Cestoda

Scientific and Common Name	Epidemiology	Disease-Producing Form and Its Location in Host	How Human Infection Occurs	Major Disease Manifestations, Diagnostic Stage, and Specimen of Choice
Echinococcus granulosus (dog tapeworm)	Worldwide in sheep-raising areas	Adult lives in the intestine of dogs or other wild canines. Larval form in human tissue causes pathology	Human accidentally ingests eggs by close contact with infected dog; usual intermediate host is sheep	Cyst can be found in the liver (most commonly) or lung of humans. Lung symptoms include coughing and pain. Leakage of hydatid fluid causes allergy and eosinophilia. Diagnosis: x ray, serology
Cysticercosis (*Taenia solium*)	Cosmopolitan	Cysticercoid larva in human tissue; usual host of larva is pig	Human accidentally ingests egg, or eggs, released from proglottid of adult in human intestine	2-cm painless swelling if in skin; pain and other symptoms if in eye; seizures or other neurologic symptoms or death if in brain
Hymenolepis diminuta (rat tapeworm)	Worldwide	Adult lives in the intestine; usual host of adult tapeworm is the rat	Human accidentally ingests cysticercoid larva in infected flea or grain beetle (intermediate host)	Mild symptoms; tapeworms are frequently lost spontaneously. Eggs in feces are diagnostic.
Dipylidium caninum (dog or cat)	Worldwide	Adult lives in the intestine; usual host of adult tapeworm is the dog or cat	Human accidentally ingests cysticercoid larva in infected dog or cat flea (intermediate host). Rare, occurs mainly in children	Mild intestinal disturbances. Tapeworms are frequently lost spontaneously. Egg packets or proglottids are diagnostic in feces.
Sparganosis (*Diphyllobothrium* or *Spirometra* spp. of dog, cat, or other mammals)	Far East freshwater areas	Plerocercoid in tissues	Human accidentally ingests copepod containing a procercoid.	Subcutaneous nodules or internal abscesses or cysts

You have now completed the section on the Cestoda. After reviewing this material and Color Plates 34–52 with the aid of your learning objectives, proceed to the post-test.

BIBLIOGRAPHY   Coltorti, EA, and Varela-Diaz, VM: Detection of antibodies against *E. granulosus* arc 5 antigens by double diffusion test. Trans R Soc Trop Med Hyg 72:227, 1978.

Leiby, PD, and Kritsky, DL: *Echinococcus multilocularis*: A possible domestic life cycle in central North America and its public health importance. J Parasitol 58:1213, 1972.

Schmidt, GD: *Handbook of Tapeworm Identification.* CRC Press, Boca Raton, FL, 1985.

Schwabe, CW, Ruppanner, R, Miller, CW, et al: Hydatid disease is endemic in California. Cal Med 117:13, 1972.

Smyth, JD: The biology of the hydatid organism. In Dawes, B (ed): *Advances in Parasitology*, Vol. 2. Academic Press, New York, 1964.

Von Bondsdorff, B: *Diphyllobothriasis in Man.* Academic Press, New York, 1977.

POST-TEST

1. Define and cite an example of each of the following: **(20 points)**
   a. Hexacanth embryo
   b. Hermaphroditic
   c. "Armed" scolex
   d. Proglottid
   e. Hydatid cyst

2. Matching: select correct intermediate host(s) for each parasite: **(10 points)**

   a. _____ *Taenia solium*

   b. _____ *Hymenolepis nana*

   c. _____ *Hymenolepis diminuta*

   d. _____ *Diphyllobothrium latum*

   e. _____ *Echinococcus granulosus*

   1. fish
   2. copepod
   3. cow
   4. human
   5. pig
   6. snail
   7. flea or beetle
   8. dog
   9. none
   10. sheep

3. Draw and label the diagnostic stage(s) for each of the following as you would observe them microscopically in human feces: **(40 points)**
   a. Dwarf tapeworm
   b. Broad fish tapeworm
   c. Beef tapeworm
   d. Pork tapeworm
   e. Hydatid cyst

4. Matching: Select one only: **(10 points)**

   a. _____ *Taenia solium*

   b. _____ *Taenia saginata*

   c. _____ *Hymenolepis nana*

   d. _____ *Diphyllobothrium latum*

   e. _____ *Echinococcus granulosus*

   f. _____ *Dipylidium caninum*

   g. _____ Sparganosis

   h. _____ Cysticercosis

   1. macrocytic anemia, vitamin B_{12} deficiency
   2. scolex lacks crown of hooks
   3. plerocercoid subcutaneously
   4. neurologic symptoms if in brain
   5. autoreinfection is common
   6. proglottid has 7 to 10 lateral uterine branches
   7. human accidentally ingests infected flea
   8. cysts found in liver, lungs, or other organs

5. A patient from the Great Lakes area presents with vague abdominal symptoms and a macrocytic anemia. Which Cestoda would be the probable cause? **(5 points)**
   a. *Diphyllobothrium latum*
   b. *Echinococcus granulosus*
   c. *Taenia saginata*
   d. *Hymenolepis nana*

6. A scolex is recovered in feces after a patient is drug-treated. The scolex bears four cup-shaped suckers. You would identify which one of the following? **(5 points)**
   a. *Diphyllobothrium latum*
   b. *Echinococcus granulosus*
   c. *Taenia saginata*
   d. *Hymenolepis nana*

7. The eggs of which two species are infective to humans if ingested, resulting in larval stages and pathology in the host's tissues? **(5 points)**
   a. *Taenia solium* and *T. saginata*
   b. *Hymenolepis diminuta* and *Dipylidium caninum*
   c. *Echinococcus granulosus* and *Taenia solium*
   d. *Hymenolepis nana* and *Taenia saginata*

8. The larval stage of which two species are infective to humans if the parasitized insect intermediate host is ingested? **(5 points)**
   a. *Taenia solium* and *T. saginata*
   b. *Hymenolepis diminuta* and *Dipylidium caninum*
   c. *Echinococcus granulosus* and *Taenia solium*
   d. *Hymenolepis nana* and *Taenia saginata*

Digenea

LEARNING OBJECTIVES

Upon completion of this chapter and its supplementary color plates as described, the student will be able to:

1 Define terminology specific for flukes.
2 State scientific and common names of flukes that parasitize humans.
3 Describe the general morphology of an adult hermaphroditic Digenea.
4 Describe the general morphology of adult schistosomes.
5 Describe graphically the life cycle of adult trematodes.
6 State the methods of diagnosis used to identify fluke infections.
7 Differentiate adult Digenea using morphologic criteria.
8 Differentiate diagnostic stages of Digenea.
9 Classify the methods by which the flukes infect humans.
10 Compare and contrast the morphology of adult Cestoda and Digenea.
11 Given an illustration or photograph (or an actual specimen if you have had laboratory experience), identify diagnostic stages of Digenea and the body specimen of choice to be used for examination of each.
12 Discriminate between the Digenea on the basis of required intermediate host(s).

Digenea (commonly called flukes) belong to the phylum Platyhelminthes along with the Cestoda. Flukes in the class Digenea (includes parasites in humans) are flattened dorsoventrally and are nonsegmented, leaf-shaped helminths. Parasitic species inhabit the intestine or tissues of humans. Digenea vary in size from a few millimeters to several centimeters in length. All adult flukes have two cup-shaped muscular suckers (**acetabula**)—an oral sucker and a ventral sucker. The digestive system is simple; the oral cavity is in the center of the oral sucker, and the intestinal tract ends blindly in one or two sacs. There is no anal opening, and waste products are regurgitated. The body surface (tegument) of the fluke is metabolically active, as is also true for the Cestoda, and can absorb soluble nutrients and release soluble waste products at the surface.

There are two types of parasitic flukes that can be present in humans. One type lives in the intestine or in other host organs, such as liver or lungs, and is hermaphroditic, having both sets of complex, highly branched reproductive organs in each adult fluke. These flukes are listed in Table 4–1. The second type are flukes that live as unisexual adult male and female organisms in the abdominal blood vessels of the definitive host. These are known as the *Schistosoma*. The body of the male schistosome curves up along the lateral edges and forms a long channel (the gynecophoral canal) that wraps around the female worm. They coexist in pairs during their adult lifespan in the blood vessels.

These flukes are listed separately in Table 4–2. In both types, sexual reproduction in the adult Digenea occurs in humans and is followed by asexual multiplication of the larval stages in a specific species of snail (a required intermediate host for all flukes).

The life cycles of the flukes are complex (see Diagram 4–1). The adult fluke lays eggs that leave the human definitive host via feces, urine, or sputum (depending upon the species and host location of the adult fluke). A specific species of freshwater snail is required as an intermediate host for each species of fluke. In general, the life cycle is as follows: the larval stage (a ciliated **miracidium**) emerges from the egg in fresh water, enters the snail host, and undergoes several cycles of asexual multiplication. The final larval stage leaving the snail is known as the **cercaria**. Many hundreds of cercariae result from asexual multiplication of each miracidium that enters the snail host. Motile schistosome (blood fluke) cercariae then directly penetrate the skin of humans when contact occurs in infected fresh water. However, the cercariae of the hermaphroditic flukes secrete a thick wall and encyst as a **metacercaria** on aquatic vegetation, or they can enter a specific second intermediate host (a freshwater fish or crustacean) and encyst. Only a few species of fish or crustaceans may serve as the second intermediate host for each species of hermaphroditic fluke. Human infection by these hermaphroditic flukes occurs, therefore, when humans eat uncooked water vegetation or the specific species of second intermediate host containing the encysted form of the larva (metacercaria).

GLOSSARY

Digenea. A class of the phylum Platyhelminthes, which includes the flukes (trematodes). These have flattened, leaf-shaped bodies bearing muscular suckers. Many species are hermaphroditic.

acetabula (sing. **acetabulum**). Muscular suckers found on the ventral surface of the flukes.

cercaria (pl. **cercariae**). The stage of the fluke life cycle that develops from germ cells in a daughter sporocyst or redia. This is the final development stage in the snail host, consisting of a body and a tail that aids in swimming after it leaves the snail.

distomiasis. Infection with flukes.

granuloma. A tumor or growth of lymphoid or other cells around a foreign body.

metacercaria (pl. **metacercariae**). The stage of the hermaphroditic fluke life cycle occurring when a cercaria has shed its tail, secreted a protective wall, and encysted as a resting stage on water plants or in a second intermediate host; infective stage for humans.

miracidium (pl. **miracidia**). Ciliated first-stage, free-swimming larva of a Digenea, which emerges from the egg and must penetrate the appropriate species of snail in order to continue its life cycle.

redia. The second or third larval stage of a trematode that develops within a sporocyst in the snail host. Elongated, saclike organisms with a mouth and a gut. Many rediae develop in one sporocyst. Each redia gives rise to many of the next trematode larval stage, the cercariae.

Schistosoma. A genus of Digenea, commonly called the blood flukes. They have an elongated shape, separate sexes, and are found in the blood vessels of their definitive host.

schistosomule. The immature schistosome in human tissues after the cercaria has lost the tail during penetration of skin.

sporocyst. The larval form of a trematode that develops from a miracidium in the snail intermediate host. It forms a simple saclike structure containing germinal cells that bud off internally and continue a process of larval multiplication, producing many rediae in each sporocyst.

Table 4-1. HERMAPHRODITIC FLUKES		
Order	**Scientific Name**	**Common Name**
Echinostomata	*Fasciolopsis buski* (fa-see′o-lop′sis/bus′kee)	large intestinal fluke
Echinostomata	*Fasciola hepatica* (fa-see′o-luh/he-pat′i-kuh)	sheep liver fluke
Opisthorchiata	*Clonorchis sinensis* (klo-nor′kis/si-nen′sis)	Chinese liver fluke
Opisthorchiata	*Heterophyes heterophyes* (het-ur-off′ee-eez/het″ur-off′ee-eez)	heterophid fluke
Opisthorchiata	*Metagonimus yokogawai* (met′uh-gon′i-mus/yo-ko-gah-wah′eye)	heterophid fluke
Plagiorchiata	*Paragonimus westermani* (par″i-gon-′i-mus/wes-tur-man′eye)	Oriental lung fluke

DIAGRAM 4–1
General life cycles of Trematoda (organ-dwelling flukes)

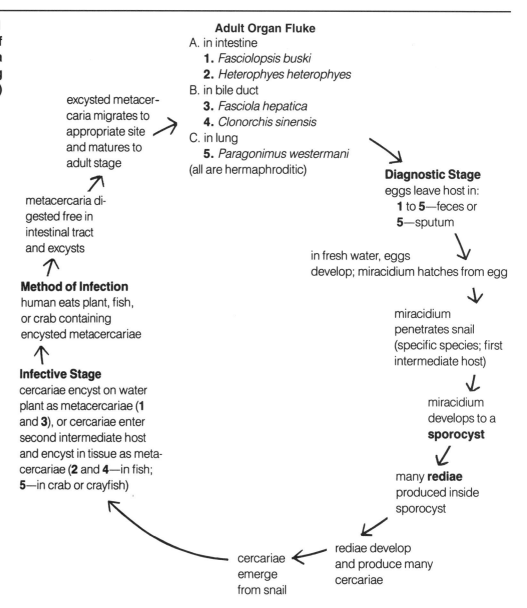

Adult Organ Fluke
A. in intestine
   1. *Fasciolopsis buski*
   2. *Heterophyes heterophyes*
B. in bile duct
   3. *Fasciola hepatica*
   4. *Clonorchis sinensis*
C. in lung
   5. *Paragonimus westermani*
(all are hermaphroditic)

excysted metacercaria migrates to appropriate site and matures to adult stage

metacercaria digested free in intestinal tract and excysts

Method of Infection
human eats plant, fish, or crab containing encysted metacercariae

Infective Stage
cercariae encyst on water plant as metacercariae (**1** and **3**), or cercariae enter second intermediate host and encyst in tissue as metacercariae (**2** and **4**—in fish; **5**—in crab or crayfish)

Diagnostic Stage
eggs leave host in:
1 to **5**—feces or
5—sputum

in fresh water, eggs develop; miracidium hatches from egg

miracidium penetrates snail (specific species; first intermediate host)

miracidium develops to a **sporocyst**

many **rediae** produced inside sporocyst

rediae develop and produce many cercariae

cercariae emerge from snail

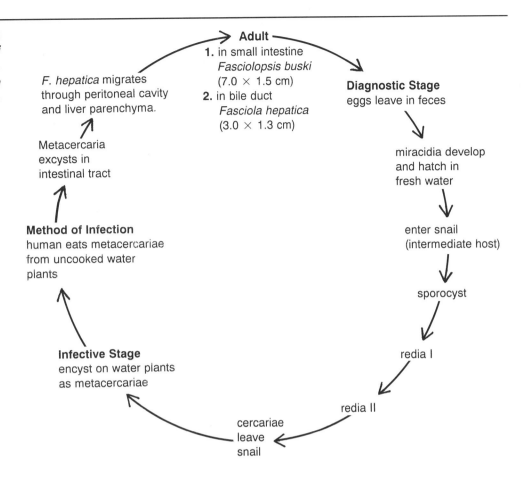

DIAGRAM 4–2
Fasciolopsis buski
(large intestinal fluke)
and *Fasciola hepatica*
(sheep liver fluke)

Adult
1. in small intestine
Fasciolopsis buski
(7.0 × 1.5 cm)
2. in bile duct
Fasciola hepatica
(3.0 × 1.3 cm)

F. hepatica migrates
through peritoneal cavity
and liver parenchyma.

Metacercaria
excysts in
intestinal tract

Method of Infection
human eats metacercariae
from uncooked water
plants

Infective Stage
encyst on water plants
as metacercariae

Diagnostic Stage
eggs leave in feces

miracidia develop
and hatch in
fresh water

enter snail
(intermediate host)

sporocyst

redia I

redia II

cercariae
leave
snail

METHOD OF DIAGNOSIS   Recovery of eggs in feces. Eggs of these two species are too similar to differentiate. Species diagnosis depends on clinical signs, travel history, and/or recovery of adult *Fasciolopis.*

DIAGNOSTIC STAGE

Egg   (*Note:* Similar for both parasites.)

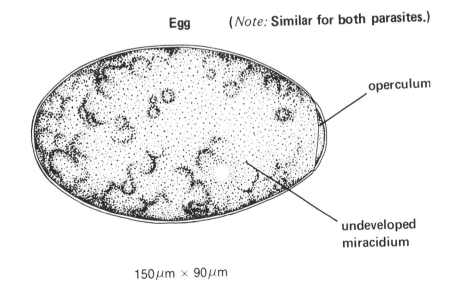

operculum

undeveloped
miracidium

150 μm × 90 μm

DISEASE NAMES   *Fasciolopis buski*—fasciolopsiasis; *Fasciola hepatica*—sheep liver rot

MAJOR PATHOLOGY AND SYMPTOMS

1. *Fasciolopsis buski*—bowel mucosal ulcers, hypersecretion and occasional hemorrhage around worm attachment site. Heavier infections cause pain, nausea, mucous diarrhea, anemia, intestinal obstruction and malabsorption, generalized edema, and marked eosinophilia; can cause death in heavy infections.
2. *Fasciola hepatica*—symptoms from mechanical irritation, toxic worm metabolites, mechanical obstruction. Migrating larvae cause local irritation. Fever, hepatomegaly, and eosinophilia in endemic areas suggest clinical diagnosis. Adults in bile duct induce portal cirrhosis in heavy infections. Jaundice, bile duct obstruction, diarrhea, and anemia may occur in severe infection. Pruritus, urticaria, cough.

TREATMENT

Fasciolopsis buski: (1) praziquantel or niclosamide, (2) tetrachloroethylene
Fasciola hepatica: bithionol

DISTRIBUTION

Fasciolopsis buski—China, Vietnam, Thailand, Indonesia, Malaysia, and the Indian subcontinent.
Fasciola hepatica—Cosmopolitan distribution in sheep- and cattle-raising countries; uncommon in the United States.

OF NOTE

1. The natural definitive host for *Fasciola hepatica* is the sheep; therefore, infection of humans is a zoonotic disease. *Fasciolopsis buski* is common in pigs.
2. *Echinostoma ilocanum* in the Philippines: 1-cm adults in small intestine; fluke has spiny collarette around oval sucker; produces eggs resembling *Fasciolopsis*. Infection results from eating raw snails.

DIAGRAM 4–3
Clonorchis sinensis (Oriental or Chinese liver fluke; *Opisthorchis*)

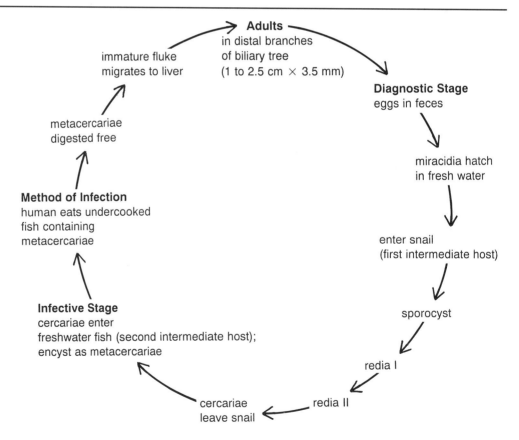

Adults
in distal branches of biliary tree
(1 to 2.5 cm × 3.5 mm)

immature fluke migrates to liver

metacercariae digested free

Method of Infection
human eats undercooked fish containing metacercariae

Infective Stage
cercariae enter freshwater fish (second intermediate host); encyst as metacercariae

Diagnostic Stage
eggs in feces

miracidia hatch in fresh water

enter snail
(first intermediate host)

sporocyst

redia I

redia II

cercariae leave snail

METHOD OF DIAGNOSIS

Recovery and identification of eggs in (1) feces or biliary drainage or from Enterotest capsule. (2) Radiographic studies.

**DIAGNOSTIC
STAGE**

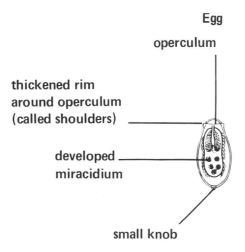

Egg

operculum

thickened rim
around operculum
(called shoulders)

developed
miracidium

small knob

30 μm × 16 μm

DISEASE NAME   Clonorchiasis

**MAJOR
PATHOLOGY AND
SYMPTOMS**

1. Light infections common and may be symptomless.
2. Jaundice because of bile duct pathology; hyperplastic changes occur.
3. Hepatomegaly with tenderness in right upper quadrant.
4. Abdominal pain and diarrhea, anorexia.
5. Chronic cases with heavy worm burden from repeated infections may induce severe hepatic complications; rarely, pancreatitis, bile duct stones, cholangitis, cholangio-carcinoma.

TREATMENT   Praziquantel

DISTRIBUTION   Far East, especially southern China

OF NOTE

1. Eggs are passed intermittently; therefore, perform repeated stool examinations.
2. Dogs and cats are reservoir hosts.

DIAGRAM 4–4
Heterophyes heterophyes and *Metagonimus yokogawai* (heterophids)

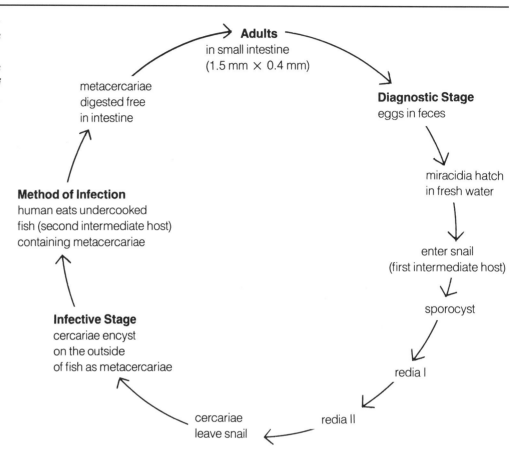

Adults
in small intestine
(1.5 mm × 0.4 mm)

metacercariae
digested free
in intestine

Diagnostic Stage
eggs in feces

Method of Infection
human eats undercooked
fish (second intermediate host)
containing metacercariae

miracidia hatch
in fresh water

enter snail
(first intermediate host)

sporocyst

Infective Stage
cercariae encyst
on the outside
of fish as metacercariae

redia I

redia II

cercariae
leave snail

METHOD OF DIAGNOSIS
Recovery and identification of eggs in feces or duodenal drainage. Difficult to differentiate. (May lack knob at end opposite operculum, which is seen on *Clonorchis sinensis* eggs.)

DIAGNOSTIC STAGE

(*Note:* **Similar for both parasites but easily confused with** *Clonorchis sinensis*.)

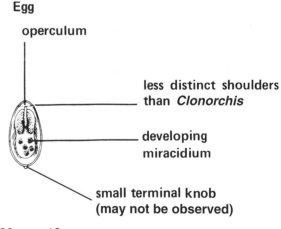

Egg
operculum

less distinct shoulders than *Clonorchis*

developing miracidium

small terminal knob (may not be observed)

30μm × 16μm

DISEASE NAMES
Heterophyes heterophyes—heterophyiasis; *Metagonimus yokogawai*—metagonimiasis

MAJOR PATHOLOGY AND SYMPTOMS
Asymptomatic unless harboring a heavy infection, which may induce a chronic mucous diarrhea and abdominal pain. Worm invasion may produce eggs that travel to heart or brain, causing symptoms of **granuloma**.

TREATMENT   Praziquantel

DISTRIBUTION   *H. heterophyes*—Near East, Far East, parts of Africa; *M. yokogawai*—Asia, including Siberia

OF NOTE   1. Primarily parasites of dogs, cats, and other fish-eating mammals.
2. Eggs may travel into tissues, causing granulomas and tissue disorders.
3. *H. heterophyes* adult has a third sucker around the genital opening.

DIAGRAM 4–5
Paragonimus westermani
(Oriental lung fluke)

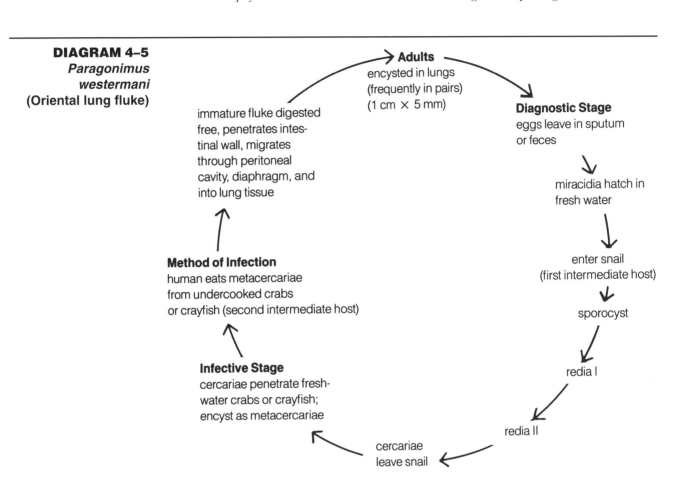

METHOD OF DIAGNOSIS   Recovery and identification of eggs in bloody sputum (resemble iron filings) or in feces; x ray of lungs showing patchy infiltrate with modular cystic shadows or calcification.

DIAGNOSTIC STAGE

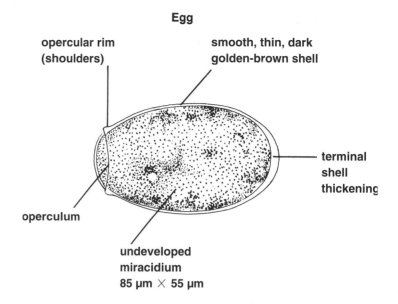

Egg

opercular rim (shoulders)

smooth, thin, dark golden-brown shell

terminal shell thickening

operculum

undeveloped miracidium
85 μm × 55 μm

DISEASE NAMES   Paragonimiasis, pulmonary **distomiasis**

MAJOR PATHOLOGY AND SYMPTOMS

1. Chronic chest pain, cough, blood-tinged sputum (rusty sputum); lung infiltration, nodules, abscesses; adults present in fibrous cysts, eggs pass through cysts and rupture into bronchioles, causing cough. Chest x ray and symptoms may resemble tuberculosis. Chronic bronchitis and increasing fibrosis.
2. Cerebral paragonimiasis causes symptoms of a space-occupying lesion. Abdominal paragonimiasis is usually asymptomatic but common.

TREATMENT

1. Praziquantel
2. Bithionol

DISTRIBUTION   Most common in the Far East; also found in parts of Africa and South America

OF NOTE

1. At least eight other species of *Paragonimus* are also infectious for humans. *P. mexicanus* in Central and South America.
2. Immature flukes may wander aberrantly to other tissues, including brain (cerebral paragonimiasis), skin, or liver.

Table 4–2. BLOOD FLUKES		
Order	**Scientific Name**	**Common Name**
Strigeata	*Schistosoma mansoni* (shis′to-so′muh/man-so′nigh)	Manson's blood fluke
Strigeata	*Schistosoma japonicum* (shis′to-so′muh/ja-pon′i-kum)	blood fluke
Strigeata	*Schistosoma haematobium* (shis′to-so′muh/hee-muh-toe′bee-um)	bladder fluke

DIAGRAM 4–6
General life cycles of
Trematoda (blood-
dwelling flukes)

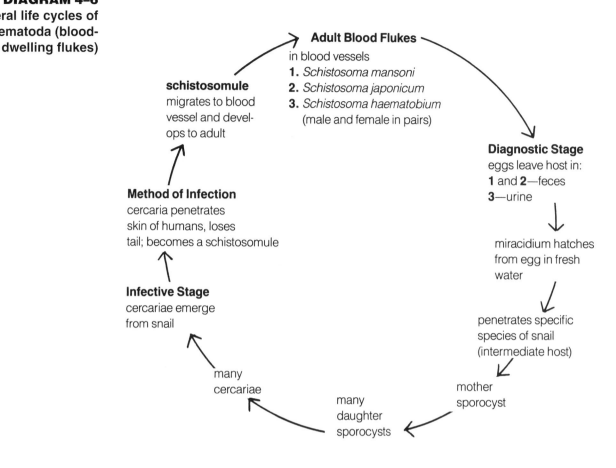

Adult Blood Flukes
in blood vessels
1. *Schistosoma mansoni*
2. *Schistosoma japonicum*
3. *Schistosoma haematobium*
(male and female in pairs)

schistosomule
migrates to blood
vessel and devel-
ops to adult

Method of Infection
cercaria penetrates
skin of humans, loses
tail; becomes a schistosomule

Infective Stage
cercariae emerge
from snail

many
cercariae

many
daughter
sporocysts

mother
sporocyst

penetrates specific
species of snail
(intermediate host)

miracidium hatches
from egg in fresh
water

Diagnostic Stage
eggs leave host in:
1 and **2**—feces
3—urine

DIAGRAM 4–7
Schistosoma **spp.**
(blood flukes)

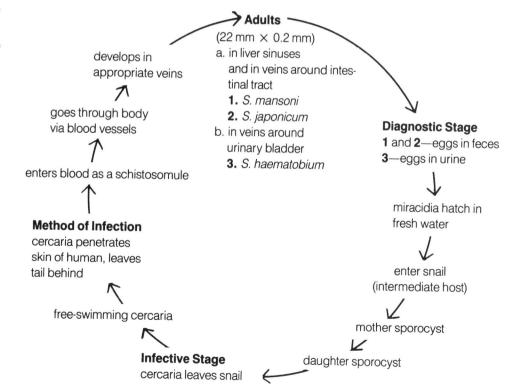

Adults
(22 mm × 0.2 mm)
a. in liver sinuses
   and in veins around intestinal tract
   1. *S. mansoni*
   2. *S. japonicum*
b. in veins around
   urinary bladder
   3. *S. haematobium*

develops in
appropriate veins

goes through body
via blood vessels

enters blood as a schistosomule

Method of Infection
cercaria penetrates
skin of human, leaves
tail behind

free-swimming cercaria

Infective Stage
cercaria leaves snail

daughter sporocyst

mother sporocyst

enter snail
(intermediate host)

miracidia hatch in
fresh water

Diagnostic Stage
1 and **2**—eggs in feces
3—eggs in urine

METHOD OF DIAGNOSIS *Schistosoma mansoni* and *S. japonicum*—recovery of eggs in feces or rectal biopsy (may require multiple biopsies for *S. mansoni*).
S. haematobium—recovery of eggs in concentrated urine.

Travel history, clinical symptoms and signs; serology; ELISA.

DIAGNOSTIC STAGES

S. mansoni **egg**

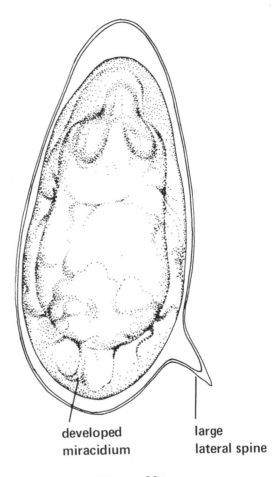

developed
miracidium

large
lateral spine

180μm × 80μm

S. japonicum **egg**

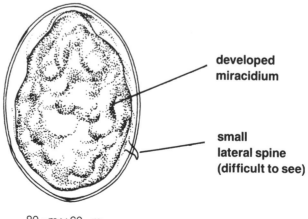

developed
miracidium

small
lateral spine
(difficult to see)

80 μm × 60 μm

S. haematobium **egg**

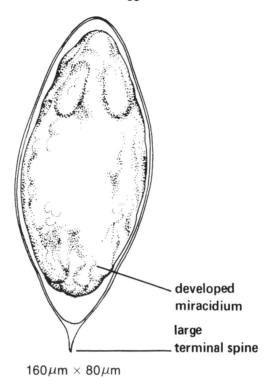

developed
miracidium

large
terminal spine

160μm × 80μm

DISEASE NAMES   Schistosomiasis, bilharziasis, swamp fever

MAJOR PATHOLOGY AND SYMPTOMS   Affects mainly children and other adults in endemic areas.

First reaction is dermatitis due to schistosome penetration.

Acute phase of first infection presents typhoid fever–like symptoms, including fever, cough, myalgias, malaise, and hepatosplenomegaly.

Cirrhosis of the liver, bloody diarrhea, bowel obstruction, hypertension, and toxic reactions because of granulomas around eggs in liver, urinary bladder, central nervous system, and other tissues. Pipestem fibrosis in liver. Infected person may develop collateral circulation if hepatic involvement is severe. Eosinophilia.

Most chronic cases are asymptomatic in endemic areas. Brown hematin pigment (identical to malarial pigment) present in phagocytic cells.

Nephrotic syndrome in *S. mansoni* and *S. haematobium.*

TREATMENT   Praziquantel

DISTRIBUTION   *S. mansoni*—Africa; South and Central America; foci in the Caribbean, including Puerto Rico and the West Indies
S. haematobium—Africa, Middle East
S. japonicum—Far East

OF NOTE   1. Schistosomiasis ranks second (behind malaria) as a cause of serious worldwide morbidity and mortality and is spreading and increasing because of recent new water-control projects, which provide increased snail breeding areas.
2. *S. haematobium* has a clinical correlation with bladder cancer.

3. Repeated infection with human or avian cercariae may induce allergic dermatitis (swimmer's itch) at freshwater swimming resorts. Occurs in North America.
4. Persistent *Salmonella* infection may be associated with *S. mansoni* and *S. japonicum.*
5. *S. intercalatum* in Africa and *S. mekongi* in the Mekong Basin.
6. *S. japonicum* infects many mammals.
7. Niclosamide lotion on the skin prevents cercarial penetration.
8. Pipestem fibrosis and collateral blood circulation may occur if liver involvement is severe.

Table 4–3. DIGENEA

Scientific and Common Name	Epidemiology	Disease-Producing Form and Its Location in Host	How Infection Occurs	Major Disease Manifestations, Diagnostic Stage, and Specimen of Choice
Fasciolopsis buski (large intestinal fluke)	Far East	Adults live in small intestine	Ingestion of encysted metacercariae on raw vegetation	Edema, eosinophilia, diarrhea, malabsorption, and even death in heavy infection. Diagnosis: eggs in feces
Fasciola hepatica (sheep liver fluke) (zoonosis)	Worldwide (in sheep- and cattle-raising areas); Humans (accidental host); Sheep (natural host)	Adults live in bile ducts	Ingestion of encysted metacercariae on raw vegetation	Traumatic tissue damage and irritation to the liver and bile ducts. Jaundice and eosinophilia can occur. Diagnosis: eggs in feces
Clonorchis sinensis (Oriental or Chinese liver fluke)	Far East	Adults live in bile ducts	Ingestion of encysted metacercariae in uncooked fish	Jaundice and eosinophilia in acute phase; long-term heavy infections lead to functional impairment of liver. Diagnosis: eggs in feces
Paragonimus westermani (Oriental lung fluke)	Far East, India, and parts of Africa	Adults live encysted in lung	Ingestion of encysted metacercariae in uncooked crab or crayfish	Chronic fibrotic disease resembling tuberculosis—cough with blood-tinged sputum. Diagnosis: egss in sputum or feces
Heterophyes heterophyes; Metagonimus yokogawai (the heterophyids)	Far East	Adults live in small intestine	Ingestion of encysted metacercariae in uncooked fish	No intestinal symptoms unless very heavy infection. Diagnosis: eggs in feces
Schistosoma mansoni (Manson's blood fluke; bilharzia; swamp fever)	Africa, Middle East, and South America	Adult in venules of the colon (eggs trapped in liver and other tissues)	Fork-tailed cercariae burrow into the capillary bed of feet, legs, or arms	Granuloma formation around eggs (i.e., in liver, intestine, and bladder). Toxic and allergic reactions; nephrotic syndrome. Diagnosis: eggs in feces; rectal biopsy
Schistosoma japonicum (Oriental blood fluke)	Far East	As above (for *Schistosoma mansoni*)	As above	As above, but symptoms are more severe due to greater egg production. Diagnosis: eggs in feces; rectal biopsy

Table 4–3. DIGENEA

Scientific and Common Name	Epidemiology	Disease-Producing Form and Its Location in Host	How Infection Occurs	Major Disease Manifestations, Diagnostic Stage, and Specimen of Choice
Schistosoma haematobium (bladder fluke)	Africa, Middle East, and Portugal	Adults in venules of bladder and rectum Eggs caught in tissues	As above	Bladder colic with blood and pus; nephrotic syndrome Systemic symptoms are mild; pulmonary involvement from eggs in lungs Has been associated with cancer of the bladder Diagnosis: eggs in urine
Swimmer's itch (zoonosis)	Worldwide	Cercariae of schistosomes that usually parasitize mammals and birds enter human skin	Fork-tailed cercariae burrow into skin of human in water	Allergic dermal response to repeated penetration (schistosomes do *not* develop to adults)

Be sure to examine Color Plates 53 to 71.

You have now completed the section on Digenea. After reviewing this material with the aid of your learning objectives, proceed to the post-test.

BIBLIOGRAPHY

Ansari, N (ed): *Epidemiology and Control of Schistosomiasis (Bilharziasis)*. University Park Press, Baltimore, 1973.

Hadden, JW, and Pascarelli, EF: Diagnosis and treatment of human fascioliasis. JAMA 202:149, 1967.

Healy GR: Trematodes transmitted to man by fish, frogs, and crustacea. J Wildl Dis 6:255, 1970.

How, PC: The relationship between primary carcinoma of the liver and infestation with *Clonorchis sinensis*. Journal of Pathology and Bacteriology 72:239, 1965.

Viranuvatti, V, and Stitnimankarn, T: Liver fluke infection and infestation in Southeast Asia. Prog Liver Dis 4:537, 1972.

Warren, KS: The pathology of schistosome infections. Helm Abstr Ser A 42:591, 1973.

Warren, KS, and Mahmoud, AAF: Algorithms in the diagnosis and management of exotic disease. I. Schistosomiasis. J Infect Dis 131:614, 1975.

Yokogawa, J: *Paragonimus* and paragonimiasis. In Dawes, B (ed): *Advances in Parasitology*. Academic Press, New York, 1969.

POST-TEST

1. Arrange these terms in order to describe the chronologic sequence of the life cycle of an intestinal trematode. **(10 points)**

   _____egg   _____metacercaria   _____miracidium   _____redia

   _____adult   _____sporocyst   _____cercaria

2. You have decided to move to the Great Lakes area of the Unites States to become a sheepherder. You will be a hermit, living a completely self-sustained life by the edge of a lake with your sheepdog and your sheep. Which of the following set of Platyhelminthes are you most likely to contract? Why did you reject each of the other answer sets? **(50 points)**
   a. *Taenia solium, Fasciola hepatica, Paragonimus westermani*
   b. *Schistosoma mansoni, Echinococcus granulosus, Clonorchis sinensis*
   c. *Fasciolopsis buski, Diphyllobothrium latum, Schistosoma japonicum*
   d. *Fasciola hepatica, Echinococcus granulosus, Diphyllobothrium latum*
   e. *Heterophyes heterophyes, Hymenolepis nana, Diphylidium caninum*

Continued

3. **(10 points)**
    a. Give the scientific and common name for each parasite represented in the following illustration of the diagnostic stage.
    b. State the method of human infection by each of the parasites represented.

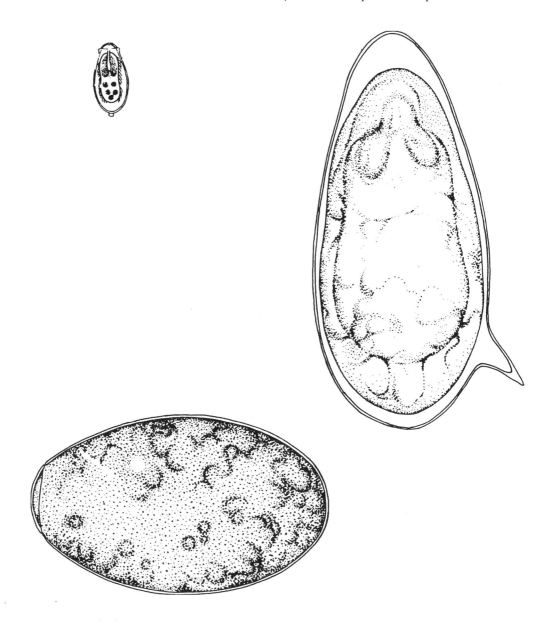

4. Why are methods of infection and control for the blood flukes different from those for the intestinal flukes? **(5 points)**

5. Humans can be infected with the larval stage of all except one of the following parasites. Which of these Digenea cannot develop as a viable larva in the tissues of humans? **(10 points)**
    a. Hydatid tapeworm   c. Pork tapeworm
    b. Bird schistosomes   d. Sheep liver fluke

6. Which of the Platyhelminthes infects humans by skin penetration and has an association with bladder cancer? **(5 points)**

7. The eggs of which flukes are undeveloped when passed in feces? **(10 points)**

Protozoa

LEARNING OBJECTIVES

Upon completion of this chapter and its supplementary color plates as described,
the student will be able to:

1   State the general characteristics of each class of **Protozoa.**
2   Define terminology specific for protozoa.
3   State the recommended methods of diagnosis of protozoal infections.
4   State any vector or intermediate host involved in the transmission of protozoal diseases.
5   Describe graphically the general life cycles for the protozoa in each class.
6   State the type of pathology caused by infection with protozoa.
7   State the scientific and common names of protozoa that parasitize humans.
8   Identify accidental protozoal infections of humans that are of medical importance.
9   Identify the type of specimen that would most likely contain the diagnostic stages of each pathogenic protozoon.
10   Discriminate between cyst and trophozoite stages of protozoa on the basis of both the morphologic criteria and the infectivity of various genera.
11   Discriminate between pathogenic and nonpathogenic amebae on the basis of morphologic criteria.
12   Differentiate species of *Plasmodium* and *Trypanosoma* by morphology and/or symptomatic criteria.
13   Discuss the medical importance of accurate identification of protozoa in humans.
14   Discuss the importance of protozoal zoonoses.
15   Discuss how the development of genetic resistance to chemicals has an impact on protozoal diseases, such as malaria.
16   Given an illustration or photograph (or an actual specimen, given sufficient laboratory experience), identify diagnostic stages of protozoa.
17   Differentiate the diagnosis of protozoa and helminths.
18   Compare and contrast life cycles of protozoa and helminths.
19   Predict the effects of immunosuppression on patients harboring various protozoal or nematode parasites.

The subkingdom Protozoa includes eukaryotic unicellular animals. The various life functions are carried out by the specialized intracellular structures known as organelles. Each group of protozoa exhibits morphologic differentiation by which it can be identified.

Most protozoa multiply by binary fission. However, certain groups have more specialized modes of reproduction that will be individually discussed.

Each species of parasitic protozoa is frequently confined to one or a few host species. At least 30 species of protozoa parasitize humans, and many of these parasitic species are widely distributed throughout the world. Other vertebrates also harbor protozoan parasites, frequently without clinical signs. Parasites that have had a long coevolution with their host species (including parasitic protozoa) have evolved adaptations that permit evasion of the host's immune recognition and response systems. It is not uncommon that accidental infection of the abnormal human host with protozoa from normal reservoir hosts causes the most serious human disease. African sleeping sickness is such an example.

There are two major methods of transmission of protozoal infection: through ingestion of the infective stage of the protozoa or by transmission via an **arthropod** vector. This is specific for each species.

The following groups are considered:
1. Amebae that move by means of **pseudopodia**
2. Protozoa that possess one to several flagella
3. Protozoa that move by means of many **cilia** on the cell surface
4. Protozoa that do not exhibit any obvious mode of mobility (This group uses sexual reproduction during the life cycle.)

Each group is listed in separate tables preceding the general discussion of each class of organisms. You should review the glossary before studying the rest of the chapter.

GLOSSARY

Protozoa. A subkingdom consisting of unicellular eukaryotic animals.

accolé. On the outer edge.

amastigote. A small, ovoid, nonflagellated form of the kinetoplastid flagellata. Notable structures include a mitochondrial kinetoplast and a large nucleus. Also called L. D. body or leishmanial form.

Apicomplexa. A phylum containing protozoa whose life cycle includes feeding stages (trophozoites), asexual multiplication (schizogony), and sexual multiplication (gametogony and sporogony).

arthropod. An organism having a hard, segmented exoskeleton and paired, jointed legs (see Chapter 6).

atria (sing. **atrium**). An opening. In a human, refers to the mouth, vagina, and urethra.

axoneme. The intracellular portion of the flagellum.

axostyle. The axial rod functioning as a support in flagellates.

blepharoplast. The basal body origin of flagella that supports the undulating membrane in kinetoplastid flagellates.

bradyzoites. Slowly multiplying intracellular trophozoites of *Toxoplasma gondii;* form cysts in immune hosts.

carrier. A host harboring and disseminating a parasite but exhibiting no clinical signs or symptoms.

chromatin. Basophilic nuclear DNA.

chromatoid body (or **bar**). A rod-shaped structure of condensed RNA material within the cytoplasm of some ameba cysts.

cilia. Hairlike processes attached to a free surface of a cell; functions for motility through fluids at the surface of the cell.

Ciliophora. A phylum containing animals that move by means of cilia and that have two dissimilar nuclei.

commensal. The association of two different species of organisms in which one partner is benefited and the other is neither benefited nor injured.

costa. A thin, firm, rodlike structure running along the base of the undulating membrane of certain flagellates.

cryptozoite. The stage of *Plasmodium* spp. that develops in liver cells from the inoculated sporozoites. Also called the exoerythrocytic stage or tissue stage.

cutaneous. Pertaining to the skin.

cyst. The immotile stage protected by a cyst wall formed by the parasite. In this stage, the protozoon is readily transmitted to a new host.

cytostome. The rudimentary mouth.

dysentery. A disorder marked by bloody diarrhea and/or mucus in feces.

ectoplasm. The gelatinous material beneath the cell membrane.

endoplasm. The fluid inner material of a cell.

endosome. The small mass of chromatin within the nucleus, comparable to a nucleolus of metazoan cells (also termed **karyosome**).

epimastigote. A flattened, spindle-shaped, flagellated form seen primarily in the gut (e.g., in the reduviid bug) or salivary glands (e.g., in the tsetse fly) of the vectors in the life cycle of trypanosomes; it has an **undulating membrane** that extends from the flagellum (attached along the anterior half of the organism) to the small kinetoplast located just anteriorly to the larger nucleus located at the midpoint of the organism.

excystation. Transformation from a cyst to a trophozoite after the cystic form has been swallowed by the host.

exflagellation. The process whereby a sporozoan microgametocyte releases haploid flagellated microgametes that can fertilize the macrogamete and thus form a diploid zygote (ookinete).

flagellum (pl. **flagella**). An extension of ectoplasm that provides locomotion; resembles a tail that moves with a whiplike motion.

fomite. An object that can adsorb and harbor organisms and can cause human infection by direct contact (e.g., wood or cloth).

gamete. A mature sex cell.

gametocyte. A sex cell that can produce gametes.

gametogony. The phase of the development cycle of the malarial and coccidial parasite in the human in which male and female gametocytes are formed.

hypnozoite. A long-surviving modified liver schizont of *P. vivax* that is the source of relapsing infections in this species.

karyosome. See **endosome.**

kinetoplast. An accessory body found in many protozoa, especially in the family Trypanosomatidae; consisting of a large mitochondrion next to the basal granule *(blepharoplast)* of the anterior or undulating membrane flagellum. Contains mitochondrial DNA.

L. D. body (Leishman-Donovan body). Each of the small ovoid amastigote forms found in tissue macrophages of the liver and spleen in patients with *Leishmania donovani* infection.

Mastigophora. A subphylum containing organisms that move by means of one or more flagella.

merogony. Asexual multiplication in coccidian life cycle. Usually occurs in intestinal epithelium.

merozoite. One of the trophozoites released from human red blood cells or liver cells at maturation of the asexual cycle of malaria.

oocyst. The encysted form of the ookinete that occurs on the stomach wall of *Anopheles* spp. mosquitoes infected with malaria.

ookinete. The motile zygote of *Plasmodium* spp.; formed by microgamete (male) fertilization of a macrogamete (female). The ookinete encysts (see **oocyst**).

paroxysm. The fever-chills syndrome in malaria. Spiking fever corresponds to the release of merozoites and toxic materials from the parasitized red blood cell (RBC), and shaking chills occur during schizont development. Occurs in malaria cyclically every 36 to 72 hours, depending on the species.

patent. Apparent or evident.

promastigote. A body similar to the epimastigote form except that the kinetoplast is located at the anterior end of the organism and therefore has no undulating membrane. This form is seen in the midgut and pharynx of vectors in the life cycle of the leishmania parasites and will be the form seen in culture media in vitro.

pseudopod. A protoplasmic extension of the trophozoites of amebae that allows them to move and to engulf food.

pseudocyst. A cystlike structure formed by the host during an acute infection with *Toxoplasma gondii.* The cyst is filled with tachyzoites in normal hosts; may occur in brain or other tissues. Latent source of infection that may become active if immunosuppression occurs.

recrudescence. A condition that may be seen in any malarial infection: infected red blood cells and accompanying symptoms reappear after a period of apparent ''cure.'' This situation reflects inadequate immune response by the host or inadequate response to treatment.

relapse (malaria). A condition seen following apparent elimination of the parasite from red blood cells; caused by a reactivation of sequestered liver merozoites that begin a new cycle in red blood cells. True relapses occur only in *P. vivax* and *P. ovale* infections.

Sarcodina. A subphylum containing amebae that move by means of pseudopodia.

schizogony (merogony). Asexual multiplication of *Apicomplexa;* multiple intracellular nuclear division precedes cytoplasmic division.

schizont. The developed stage of asexual division of the *Sporozoa* trophozoite (e.g., *Plasmodium* spp. in a human red blood cell, *Isospora belli* in the intestinal wall).

sporocyst. The fertilized oocyst in which the sporozoites of *Plasmodium* have developed.

sporogony. Sexual reproduction of *Apicomplexa.* Production of spores and sporozoites.

sporozoite. The form of *Plasmodium* that develops inside the sporocyst, invades the salivary glands of the mosquito, and is transmitted to humans.

subpatent. Not evident, subclinical.

tachyzoites. Rapidly growing intracellular trophozoites of *Toxoplasma gondii.*

trophozoite (pl. **trophozoites**). The motile stage of protozoon that feeds, multiplies, and maintains the colony within the host.

trypomastigote. A body similar to the epimastigote form except that the kinetoplast is located at the posterior end of the organism and the undulating membrane extends along the entire body from the flagellum (anterior end) to the posterior end at the blepharoplast. This form is seen in the blood of humans with trypanosomiasis and as the infective stage in the insect vectors.

undulating membrane. A protoplasmic membrane with a flagellar rim extending out like a fin along the outer edge of the body of certain protozoa; it moves in a wavelike pattern.

xenodiagnosis. Infections with *Trypanosoma cruzi* may be diagnosed by allowing an uninfected *Triatoma* bug to feed on the patient (the bite is painless); the insect's feces are later examined for parasites (trypanosome forms).

zygote. The fertilized cell resulting from the union of male and female gametes.

CLASS LOBOSEA

Amebae in the order Amoebida (Table 5–1), which are parasites of humans, can be found worldwide. The motile, reproducing feeding stage (the **trophozoite**) lives most commonly in the lower gastrointestinal tract. Many of these amebae can form a nonfeeding, nonmotile **cyst** stage, which is the stage that is infective for humans. Transmission of amebae is generally by ingestion of cysts in fecally contaminated food or water. When cysts are swallowed and pass to the lower intestine, they **excyst** and begin to multiply as feeding **trophozoites.**

The structure of the nucleus is quite different for each genus of ameba, and identification of nuclear structure aids in diagnosis. A permanent stain such as the trichrome stain used on a thin, fixed fecal smear is particularly helpful in identifying nuclear structures and is highly recommended as a routine procedure in a diagnostic laboratory. Other diagnostic features include size, cytoplasmic inclusions, and type of motility exhibited by the pseudopodia formed by trophozoites in a wet-mount preparation. In the

Table 5–1. AMEBAE

Order	Scientific Name	Common Name
Amoebida	*Entamoeba histolytica* (en'tuh-mee'buh/his-toe-lit'i-kuh)	Amebic dysentery
Amoebida	*Entamoeba hartmanni* (en'tuh-mee'buh/hart-man'nee)	Small race of *E. histolytica*
Amoebida	*Entamoeba coli* (en'tuh-mee'buh/ko'lye)	Commensal
Amoebida	*Entamoeba polecki* (en'tuh-mee'buh/po-lek'ee)	Commensal
Amoebida	*Entamoeba gingivalis* (en'tuh-mee'buh/gin-gi-val'is)	Commensal
Amoebida	*Blastocystis hominis* (blast'o-sis-tis/hom-in'is)	Commensal
Amoebida	*Endolimax nana* (en'doe-lye'macks/nay'nuh)	Commensal
Amoebida	*Iodamoeba bütschlii* (eye-o'duh-mee'buh/bootch'lee-eye)	Commensal
Amoebida	*Acanthamoeba* spp. (ay-kanth'uh-mee'buh)	None
Schizopyrenida	*Naegleria fowleri* (nay'gleer-ee'uh fow-ler'i)	Primary amebic meningoencephalitis

cyst stage, nuclear structure, the size and shape of the cyst, the number of nuclei, and other inclusion bodies present are diagnostic features.

Entamoeba histolytica is the major pathogen in this group and is the cause of amebic dysentery in humans. It can occur in other primates, dogs, cats, and rats. All other amebae seen in feces are considered to be nonpathogenic **commensals**. It is important, however, that each species be correctly identified to ensure proper therapy, if needed, and to avoid unnecessary treatment owing to misdiagnosis.

The nucleus of *E. histolytica* has a small central **karyosome (endosome)** and uniform peripheral chromatin granules lining the nuclear membrane. *E. histolytica* invades the intestinal wall and multiplies in the mucosal tissue. In the cytoplasm of the trophozoite, one can frequently see ingested red blood cells; the trophozoite voraciously feeds on these red blood cells when it is invasive. The red blood cells can appear either whole or partially digested. These blood cells are not seen in the trophozoite of any other ameba, and their presence helps in differential diagnosis. The trophozoite of *E. histolytica* extends thin pseudopodia and exhibits active, progressive motility in a wet mount.

The cyst of *E. histolytica* contains one, two, or four nuclei: Nuclear divisions accompany cyst maturation. The nuclear structure, as seen in stained cysts or in trophozoites, is the same.

The cyst of the pathogenic *E. histolytica* is round and is 10 to 20 μm in size. It may also contain cigar-shaped **chromatoid bars.** A small race of *E. histolytica* is nonpathogenic and may be confused with *Entamoeba hartmanni*, which forms cysts of less than 10 μm and is also nonpathogenic. A calibrated ocular micrometer (see page 125) is required to measure cyst diameters. Pathology caused by *E. histolytica* includes flask-shaped ulcerations of the intestinal wall and bloody dysentery. If amebae penetrate the intestinal wall and spread via blood, ulceration may occur in the liver, lungs, brain, or other tissues. This can be fatal. Prevalence is very high in the subtropics and tropics (over 50 percent), and focal epidemics can occur anywhere. Prevalence in the United States and Europe is around 5 percent, with most being **carriers.**

Entamoeba coli (a nonpathogenic commensal) is most commonly confused with *E. histolytica*. The nucleus of *E. coli* differs from *E. histolytica;* it has a large eccentric karyosome and irregular peripheral chromatin clumping along the nuclear membrane. The trophozoite exhibits granular cytoplasm and ingested bacteria but not red blood cells. Motility is sluggish. The cyst stage often has up to eight nuclei of characteristic structure rather than a maximum of four as in *E. histolytica*. Chromatoid bars, if present, have pointed rather than rounded ends.

Entamoeba polecki, found primarily in pigs and monkeys, is occasionally found in humans. It closely resembles both *E. histolytica* and *E. coli* morphologically. Great care is needed when identifying this organism because it is not pathogenic, and unnecessary treatment results if it is incorrectly differentiated as *E. histolytica.* This organism is identified by noting the usual one nucleus in mature cysts. Rarely, there may be two or four nuclei. A large glycogen "inclusion mass" may also be present. Chromatoid bodies are abundant and are pointed rather than rounded as in *E. histolytica.*

Entamoeba gingivalis, found in the mouth in soft tartar between teeth or in tonsillar crypts, is considered nonpathogenic but can occasionally be found in sputum and must be diffentiated from *E. histolytica.* Two important features help in this regard: *E. gingivalis* has no cyst stage, and it is the only species known to ingest white blood cells. Nuclear fragments of white cells can be seen in the trophozoite's large food vacuoles when permanently stained smears are examined.

Blastocystis hominis is a strictly anaerobic intestinal protozoon that has been variously classified since its discovery in 1912. It multiplies by binary fission or sporulation. Fecal-oral transmission through contaminated food or water is probably the route of infection. This parasite generally does not seem to cause clinical disease in humans but must be considered when found in large numbers in patients with abdominal symptoms who have no other apparent etiologic agent. Metronidazole (Flagyl) is the drug of choice when treatment is needed.

When present, *B. hominis* are easily recovered and are identified using the trichrome stain. The organism is round and varies greatly in size from 6 to 40 μm in diameter. The central area of the cell resembles a large vacuole surrounded by several small dark-staining nuclei. These organisms may be confused with yeast cells. When processing fecal samples, only saline should be used to wash the specimen because water destroys *B. hominis,* causing a false-negative report.

Cysts of amebae may have varying numbers of nuclei, depending on their stage of development; therefore, it is critical to look at nuclear structure as well as numbers for identification. Additionally, *Dientamoeba fragilis* (a flagellate) may occasionally have more or fewer than two nuclei in the trophozoite stage and could therefore be confused with developing cysts of *Endolimax nana* or other ameba.

Several species of free-living amebae may become opportunistic parasites of humans. These organisms are found in fresh or salt water, moist soil, and decaying vegetation. In most instances, no disease is produced by these organisms, but in a few cases, severe consequences result. The notable potential pathogens are *Naegleria fowleri* and, less commonly, *Acanthamoeba* spp. *Naegleria* is actually an ameboflagellate, because in the free-living state it alternates from an ameboid phase to a form possessing two flagella. Only the ameboid phase is found in host tissues.

The disease caused by *N. fowleri* occurs most often during the summer months. The parasite gains entry through the nasal mucosa when the host is diving and swimming in ponds or small lakes that are inhabited by the parasite. This parasite tolerates chlorinated water and has even been found in an indoor swimming pool. Furthermore, infections have been acquired by drinking unfiltered, chlorinated tap water. Upon infection, the clinical symptoms are very dramatic, and the disease runs a very rapid and usually fatal course. Symptoms of primary amebic meningoencephalitis (PAM) begin with headache, fever, nausea, and vomiting within 1 or 2 days. Typical symptoms of meningoencephalitis follow, leading to irrational behavior, coma, and death. The clinical course rarely lasts more than 6 days.

Diagnosis is often made on autopsy; however, a purulent spinal fluid containing high numbers of neutrophils (200 to 20,000/μl) without bacteria should add amebic meningoencephalitis to the differential diagnosis. Motile amebae may be noted in unstained preparations. A drop of unrefrigerated spinal fluid sediment should be examined on a clean glass slide for motility because the organism resembles a leukocyte when observed on a counting chamber. Phase microscopy is preferred, but the motile trophozoite may be observed using a bright-field microscope with reduced light. Giemsa or Wright stain is helpful. Its ameboid form is elongated with a tapered posterior and ranges from 7 to 20 μm. The rounded form is 15 μm with a large central nuclear karyosome and granular, vacuolated cytoplasm. Treatment is usually unsuccessful; however, amphotericin B and sulfadiazine have been effective in a very few cases when given promptly.

Acanthamoeba spp. cause a more chronic form of meningoencephalitis, granulomatous amebic encephalitis (GAE). Infected patients frequently have compromised immunologic systems. Onset of symptoms is slow, usually 10 days or more. Chronic granulomatous lesions in brain tissue may contain both trophozoites and cysts. These parasites have been found in lungs, nasal passages, eyes, ears, skin lesions, and the vagina. There have also been several hundred cases of acanthamoeba keratitis related to poor contact lens care.

Cysts of *Acanthamoeba* spp., like *Naegleria* spp., are also resistant to chlorination and drying. The parasite may be transported by water and possibly through air. *Acanthamoeba* spp. trophozoites have spinelike pseudopodia but are rarely seen motile. They average 30 μm and have a large central karyosome in the nucleus. The cyst is round with a single nucleus and a double cyst wall; the outer cyst wall may be slightly wrinkled with a polyhedral inner wall. *Acanthamoeba* spp. vary in sensitivity to antimicrobial agents.

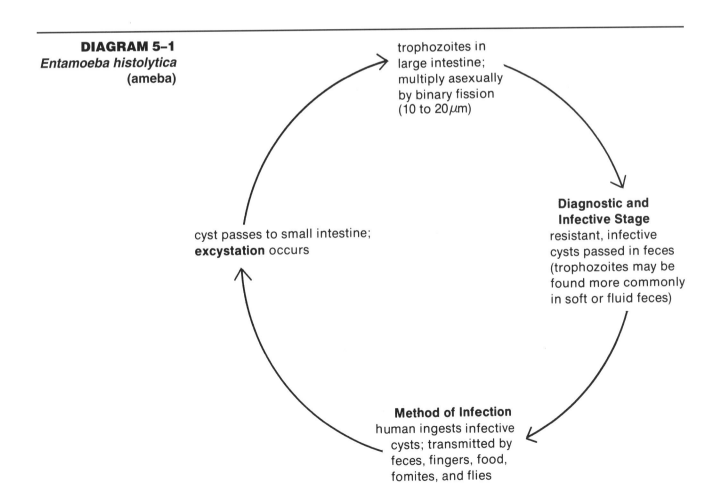

DIAGRAM 5–1
Entamoeba histolytica
(ameba)

trophozoites in large intestine; multiply asexually by binary fission (10 to 20 μm)

Diagnostic and Infective Stage
resistant, infective cysts passed in feces (trophozoites may be found more commonly in soft or fluid feces)

Method of Infection
human ingests infective cysts; transmitted by feces, fingers, food, fomites, and flies

cyst passes to small intestine; **excystation** occurs

METHOD OF DIAGNOSIS   Recovery and identification of trophozoites or cysts in feces or intestinal mucosa

SPECIMEN REQUIREMENTS
1. At least three fresh stool specimens should be examined for the presence of parasites. A permanently stained smear and a saline mount of each specimen should be prepared and examined.
2. Six permanent smears from different sites should be prepared while a sigmoidoscopy is being performed.
3. Serologic methods are most useful in extraintestinal diseases.

DIAGNOSTIC STAGE

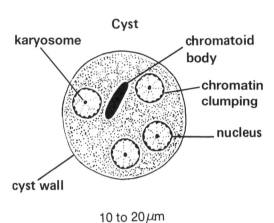

Cyst

karyosome

chromatoid body

chromatin clumping

nucleus

cyst wall

10 to 20 μm

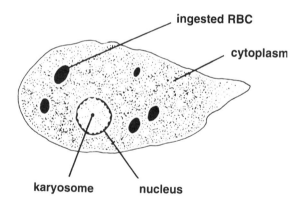

Trophozoite

ingested RBC

cytoplasm

karyosome   nucleus

10 to 20 μm

Note: Even pattern of nuclear chromatin on the nuclear rim with spokelike pattern from the karysome.

DISEASE NAMES   Amebiasis, amebic dysentery, amebic hepatitis (if liver is involved)

MAJOR PATHOLOGY AND SYMPTOMS   May be asymptomatic or exhibit vague abdominal discomfort, malaise, diarrhea alternating with constipation, or, if acute, bloody dysentery and fever. Invades intestinal submucosa via lytic enzymes in 2 to 8 percent of infections; lateral extension leads to typical flask-shaped lesions. In amebic hepatitis there is an enlarged liver, fever, chills, and leukocytosis.

TREATMENT Depends on location of infection: iodoquinol, paromomycin, metronidazole, dehydroemetine, and combinations (see *Medical Letter* items in Bibliography on page 157). All positive cases should be treated.

DISTRIBUTION Worldwide

OF NOTE
1. Chronic infection may last for years.
2. Recent studies indicate that the pathogenic and a nonpathogenic strain of *E. histolytica* can be differentiated definitively only by using DNA probes.
3. Onset of invasive disease may be gradual or sudden and is characterized by blood-tinged mucous dysentery with up to 10 stools per day. Severe, sudden-onset cases may mimic appendicitis.
4. Must be differentiated from ulcerative colitis, carcinoma, other intestinal parasites, and diverticulitis. Also, the hepatic form must be differentiated from hepatitis, hydatid cyst, various gallbladder problems, cancer, and lung disease.
5. Ameba can invade lungs, brain, skin, and other tissues. Hepatic amebiasis is the most common and gravest complication. Usually only a single abscess develops in the right lobe of the liver. Any of the various imaging techniques reveals the abscess.
6. This parasite has been added to the list of sexually transmitted diseases.

Comparative Morphology of Intestinal Amebae

                                    Cyst   Trophozoite

Entamoeba histolytica

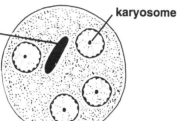

chromatoid body   **karyosome**   **Red blood cells being digested**

Note: identical nuclear morphology in cyst and trophozoite

diameter over 10 μm, up to 4 nuclei in cyst,
central karyosome, even nuclear chromatin at edges,
and spokelike rays of chromatin from karyosome outward;
chromatoid body has blunt, rounded ends that are
noted more frequently than those seen in *E. coli* cysts;
precysts may have a glycogen vacuole that stains reddish-brown

                    Cyst   **Trophozoite**

Entamoeba hartmanni (small race of
E. histolytica; nonpathogenic)

                        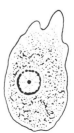

            diameter less than 10 μm   *Continued*

Cyst   **Trophozoite**

Entamoeba coli

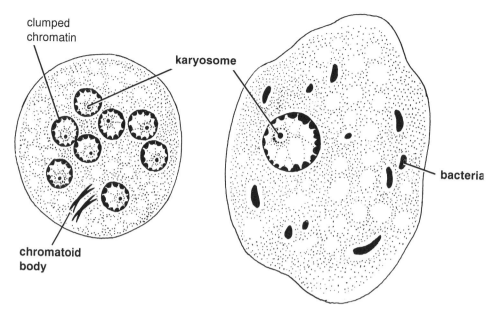

clumped
chromatin

karyosome

**chromatoid
body**

bacteria

A   diameter over 10 μm, up to 8 nuclei in cyst;
eccentric karyosome, irregular, clumped nuclear chromatin;
when present, chromatoid body is
splinter-shaped with rough pointed edges   B

Cyst   **Trophozoite**

Endolimax nana

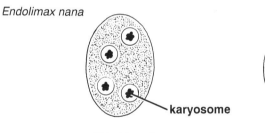

karyosome

(6 to 12 μm)
up to 4 nuclei in cyst;
large irregular karyosome
no peripheral chromatin,
cyst has ovoid shape

Cyst   **Trophozoite**

Iodamoeba bütschlii

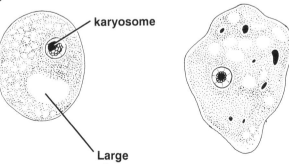

karyosome

**Large
glycogen
vacuole**

(8 to 10 μm)
single nucleus
large irregular karyosome
no peripheral chromatin

(stains brown with iodine)

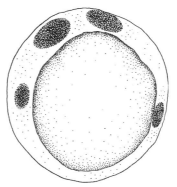

Blastocystis hominis
5 to 30 μm

Cyst

Trophozoite

Naegleria fowleri

no cyst present
in tissue

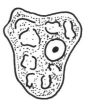

7 to 20 μm

Cyst

Trophozoite

Acanthamoeba spp.

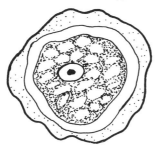

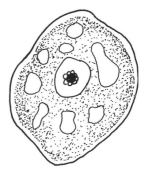

15 to 20 μm

10 to 45 μm

cyst present in tissue;
has a wrinkled
double wall

large round trophozoite
with a distinct nucleus
and smooth-staining
cytoplasm when viewed
in tissue

SUPERCLASS MASTI-GOPHORA Flagellates in the class Zoomastigophorea include the pathogenic protozoa that inhabit the gastrointestinal tract, **atria,** bloodstream, or tissues of humans. The parasites considered in this group are listed in Table 5–2. The pathogenic intestinal flagellates include only two of the species, *Giardia lamblia* and *Dientamoeba fragilis.* Two common nonpathogenic species found in the intestinal tract include *Chilomastix mesnili* and *Trichomonas hominis.* These organisms must be differentiated from pathogens to avoid misdiagnosis

Order	Scientific Name	Common Name
	Table 5-2. FLAGELLATES	
Diplomonadida	*Giardia lamblia* (gee'are-dee'uh/lamb-blee'uh)	traveler's diarrhea
Trichomonadida	*Dientamoeba fragilis* (dye-en'tuh-mee'buh/fradj"i-lis)	*Dientamoeba*
Trichomonadida	*Trichomonas vaginalis* (trick"o-mo'nas/vadj-i-nay'lis)	trich
Kinetoplastida	*Trypanosoma brucei rhodesiense* (trip-an"o-so"muh/brew'see"i/ro-dee"zee-en'see)	East African sleeping sickness
Kinetoplastida	*Trypanosoma brucei gambiense* (trip-an"o-so'muh/brew'see"i/gam-bee-en'see)	West African sleeping sickness
Kinetoplastida	*Trypanosoma cruzi* (trip-an"o-so'muh/kroo'zye)	Chagas' disease
Kinetoplastida	*Leishmania tropica* complex (leesh-may'nee-uh/trop'i-kuh)	Oriental boil
Kinetoplastida	*Leishmania mexicana* complex (leesh-may'nee-uh/mex-i-can'uh)	New World leishmaniasis
Kinetoplastida	*Leishmania braziliensis* complex (leesh-may'nee-uh/bra-zil"i-en'sis)	New World leishmaniasis
Kinetoplastida	*Leishmania donovani* complex (leesh-may'nee-uh/don"o-vay'nigh)	kala-azar

and mistreatment. There is only one pathogenic atrial protozoan—*Trichomonas vaginalis*—that inhabits the vagina and urethra. In the order Kinetoplastida, two genera are pathogenic and multiply in the tissues of humans. These are the genus *Trypanosoma,* which has three major pathogenic species, and the genus *Leishmania,* which has four major pathogenic species.

Giardia lamblia is the most common intestinal parasite in the United States. Of the intestinal flagellates, it is important to differentiate *G. lamblia* from the several nonpathogenic flagellates that can be found in the intestinal tract. The trophozoite and the cyst are illustrated on page 75. The trophozoite of *G. lamblia* (10 to 20 μm $\times$ 5 to 15 μm) is bilaterally symmetric and has two anterior nuclei and eight **flagella.** A sucking disk concavity on the ventral side is the means of attachment to the intestinal mucosa. The cysts are oval, with two or four nuclei located at one end. The clustered nuclei and the central **axoneme** give the cyst the appearance of "a little old lady wearing glasses." The cytoplasm is often retracted from the cyst wall, leaving a clear space under the wall. This parasite has frequently been associated with traveler's diarrhea, and both trophozoites and cysts can be found in the diarrheic feces along with unusual amounts of mucus. These are not tissue invaders; however, prolonged heavy infection may result in malabsorption by the intestinal mucosa. Transmission is by ingestion of the cyst stage in fecally contaminated water or food.

Dientamoeba fragilis also has been associated with cases of diarrhea. It lives in the cecum and colon and does not form cysts; the method of transmission is uncertain. The trophozoite has two nuclei connected by a division spindle filament. It has no observable flagella but is classified as a trichomonad even though it moves by means of pseudopodia rather than flagella when seen in feces. The trophozoite is 6 to 20 μm and exhibits sluggish nondirectional motility.

Trichomonas vaginalis multiplies in the genitourinary atrium of both males and females. Usually only females exhibit symptoms, and males serve as asymptomatic **carriers.** Transmission of *T. vaginalis* is generally by sexual intercourse. Trichomonad species do not form cysts. Motile trophozoites may be identified in fresh urine or in a urethral or vaginal smear by its characteristic structure. It has a large anterior nucleus, four anterior flagella, an **axostyle,** and an **undulating membrane.** Even though the male is usually asymptomatic, all sex partners should be treated so that reinfection of the female partner does not recur.

In the order Kinetoplastida, the pathogenic *Trypanosoma* and *Leishmania* flagellates multiply in the blood (hemoflagellates) or tissue of humans. All species require an arthropod intermediate host. Furthermore, the hemoflagellates exhibit specific morphology in specific locations in both humans and arthropods.

In the genus *Trypanosoma,* two subspecies, *T. brucei rhodesiense* and *T. brucei gambiense,* cause East and West African sleeping sickness, respectively. These diseases are transmitted by the tsetse fly intermediate host (*Glossina* spp.). Organisms are injected when the infected fly takes a blood meal. The **trypomastigote** form can be found in a human blood smear extracellularly in the plasma or in tissues such as lymph node biopsies or in the central nervous system late in the disease.

The species *T. cruzi,* primarily found in Central and South America, causes a debilitating condition known as Chagas' disease. *T. cruzi* is transmitted by the *Triatoma* bug intermediate host. When the *Triatoma* takes a blood meal, infective organisms are deposited on the skin (in the feces of the bug) and are rubbed into the wound when the itching bite site is scratched. *T. cruzi* organisms multiply in macrophages of the reticuloendothelial system and are found multiplying as the **amastigote** form in tissues such as the heart. However, trypomastigote forms may be found in the bloodstream early during the infection. Chagas' disease can result in enlarged heart, esophagus, and colon, and eventually in death, if untreated. In children, an acute fatal disease course is not uncommon.

In the genus *Leishmania,* there are four pathogenic ''species complexes'' with subspecies in each complex: *L. tropica* (Old World), *L. mexicana* (New World), *L. braziliensis,* and *L. donovani.* Speciation has traditionally been based on clinical symptomology, geographic location, and case history. All *Leishmania* species are transmitted by the sandfly intermediate host *Phlebotomus* spp. The bite of an infected sandfly results initially in a self-healing lesion of the skin at the bite site, which may last up to a year and may be a wet or dry ulcer, depending on the species. Amastigote forms can be found multiplying intracellularly in local macrophages of the lesion. *L. tropica* and *L. mexicana* cause cutaneous, spontaneously healing ulcers, although some subspecies of *L. mexicana* spread to cause disfiguring diffuse cutaneous leishmaniasis (DCL). *L. braziliensis* affects the mucosa of the nasopharynx and mouth. Additionally, *L. braziliensis* can become **subpatent** and flare up years later, resulting in erosion of cartilage in the nose and ears.

Unlike the others, *L. donovani* does not stay localized in the skin lesion; the organisms spread to the viscera, multiplying in macrophages of all internal organs and eventually causing death if the patient is untreated. In tissue sections (e.g., liver or spleen), *L. donovani* can be seen as intracellular multiplying amastigote forms **(L.D. bodies)**. All species of *Leishmania* that infect humans are zoonotic; the usual host is a vertebrate such as a dog, fox, or rodent.

DIAGRAM 5–2
Giardia lamblia
(flagellate)

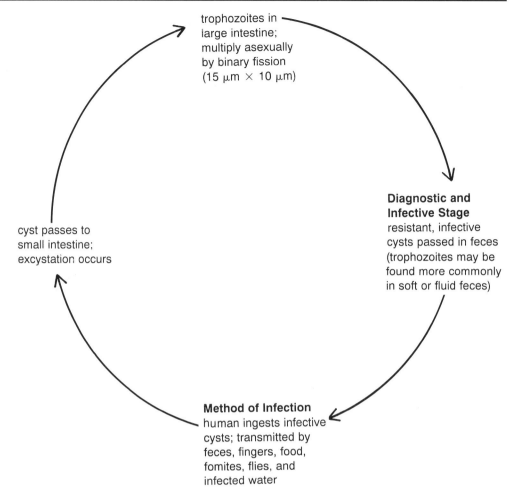

trophozoites in
large intestine;
multiply asexually
by binary fission
(15 μm × 10 μm)

**Diagnostic and
Infective Stage**
resistant, infective
cysts passed in feces
(trophozoites may be
found more commonly
in soft or fluid feces)

cyst passes to
small intestine;
excystation occurs

Method of Infection
human ingests infective
cysts; transmitted by
feces, fingers, food,
fomites, flies, and
infected water

**METHOD OF
DIAGNOSIS**
Recovery and identification of trophozoites or cysts in feces or duodenal contents*

**SPECIMEN
REQUIREMENTS**
1. At least three stool specimens should be examined for possible parasites.
2. A permanently stained smear for each specimen should be prepared and examined.
3. Be sure to examine areas of mucus for the possible presence of parasites.

---

*A commercially available, orally retrievable string device (swallowed in a gelatin capsule)—Enterotest (available from "Hedeco," Health Development Corp., East Palo Alto, CA)—can be examined for the presence of trophozoites in duodenal mucus adherent on the string, which is pulled up after capsule has been swallowed. The device is also useful for recovering *Strongyloides stercoralis* eggs and/or larvae.

DIAGNOSTIC STAGE

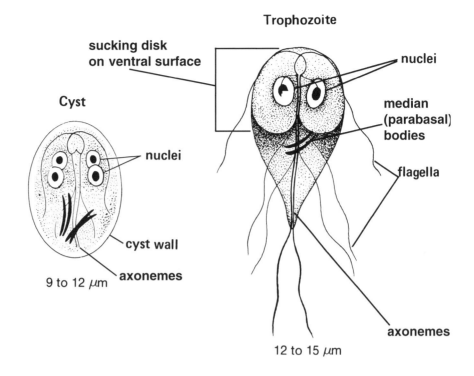

Trophozoite

sucking disk on ventral surface

nuclei

median (parabasal) bodies

flagella

axonemes

12 to 15 μm

Cyst

nuclei

cyst wall

axonemes

9 to 12 μm

DISEASE NAMES	Giardiasis, traveler's diarrhea
MAJOR PATHOLOGY AND SYMPTOMS	Abdominal pain, foul-smelling diarrhea, foul-smelling gas (known as the "purple burps"; smells like rotten eggs), mechanical irritation of intestinal mucosa with shortening of villi and inflammatory foci; malabsorption syndrome in heavy infections. Persons with an immunoglobulin class A deficiency may be more susceptible. Stool does not contain red or white blood cells as in bacillary dysentery.
TREATMENT	1. Quinacrine 2. Metronidazole or furazolidone
DISTRIBUTION	Worldwide
OF NOTE	1. Recent outbreaks have been related to cross-contamination of water and sewage systems as well as to wild animals such as beavers that serve as reservoir hosts. 2. Travelers to endemic areas (such as St. Petersburg in Russia and some American areas as well) experience severe diarrhea upon infection, but permanent residents of the endemic areas generally do not.

DIAGRAM 5–3
Dientamoeba fragilis
(intestinal flagellate)

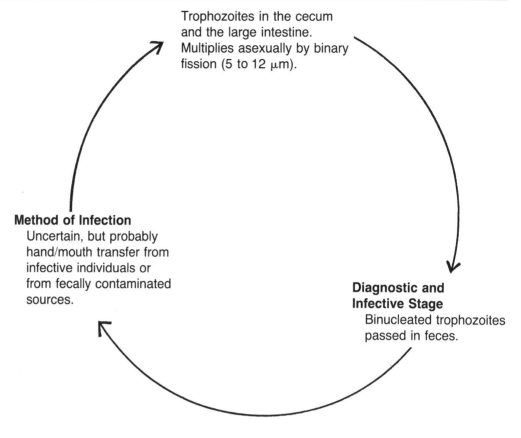

Trophozoites in the cecum and the large intestine. Multiplies asexually by binary fission (5 to 12 μm).

Method of Infection
Uncertain, but probably hand/mouth transfer from infective individuals or from fecally contaminated sources.

Diagnostic and Infective Stage
Binucleated trophozoites passed in feces.

METHOD OF DIAGNOSIS   Identification of trophozoites in feces (no cyst stage known)

SPECIMEN REQUIREMENTS
1. At least three stool specimens should be examined for parasites.
2. A permanently stained smear for each specimen should be prepared and examined, especially because there is no cyst stage.
3. Trophozoites can be found in formed stools.

DIAGNOSTIC STAGE

Dientamoeba fragilis   **(two nuclei)**

No cyst stage known

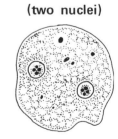

MAJOR PATHOLOGY AND SYMPTOMS   Usually asymptomatic; may be associated with diarrhea, anorexia, abdominal pain

TREATMENT   Iodoquinol, tetracycline, or paromomycin

DISTRIBUTION   Worldwide

OF NOTE   1. A fairly high association between *Enterobius vermicularis* and *D. fragilis* infections has been noted. These findings suggest that *D. fragilis* may also be transmitted via pinworm eggs.
2. No cyst stage is known for this parasite.
3. Most organisms have two nuclei.

Nonpathogenic Intestinal Flagellates

Chilomastix mesnili

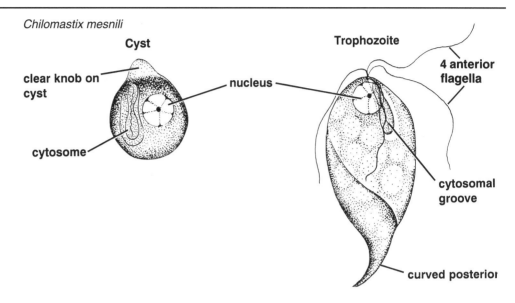

Cyst

clear knob on cyst

cytosome

nucleus

Trophozoite

4 anterior flagella

cytosomal groove

curved posterior

Trichomonas hominis

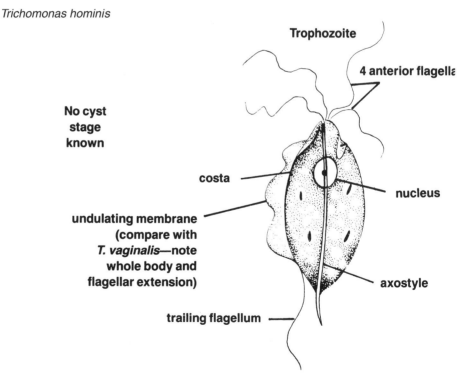

Trophozoite

No cyst stage known

4 anterior flagella

costa

nucleus

undulating membrane (compare with *T. vaginalis*—note whole body and flagellar extension)

axostyle

trailing flagellum

DIAGRAM 5-4
Trichomonas vaginalis (atrial flagellate)

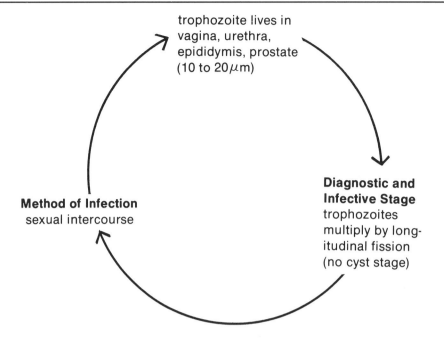

trophozoite lives in vagina, urethra, epididymis, prostate (10 to 20 μm)

Diagnostic and Infective Stage
trophozoites multiply by long-itudinal fission (no cyst stage)

Method of Infection
sexual intercourse

METHOD OF DIAGNOSIS   Recovery and identification of motile trophozoites in a fresh urethral discharge, vaginal smear, or urine. Can be recognized in Papanicolaou-stained cervical smear.

SPECIMEN REQUIREMENTS
1. Fresh vaginal or urethral discharges or prostatic secretions are examined as a wet mount diluted with a drop of saline.
2. Several specimens may be needed before diagnosis is confirmed.

DIAGNOSTIC STAGE

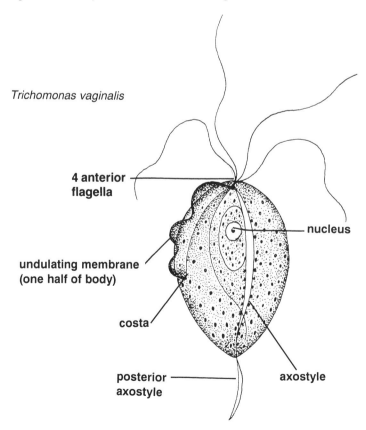

Trichomonas vaginalis

4 anterior flagella

nucleus

undulating membrane (one half of body)

costa

posterior axostyle

axostyle

Trophozoite (no cyst stage form)
15 μm

DISEASE NAMES Trichomonad vaginitis, urethritis, trich

MAJOR PATHOLOGY AND SYMPTOMS
1. Female:
   a. Persistent vaginal inflammation
   b. Yellowish, frothy, foul-smelling vaginal discharge
   c. Burning urination
   d. Itching and irritation
2. Male: generally asymptomatic

TREATMENT Metronidazole

DISTRIBUTION Worldwide

DIAGRAM 5–5
Trypanosoma brucei rhodesiense (East African sleeping sickness) and *Trypanosoma brucei gambiense* (West African sleeping sickness)

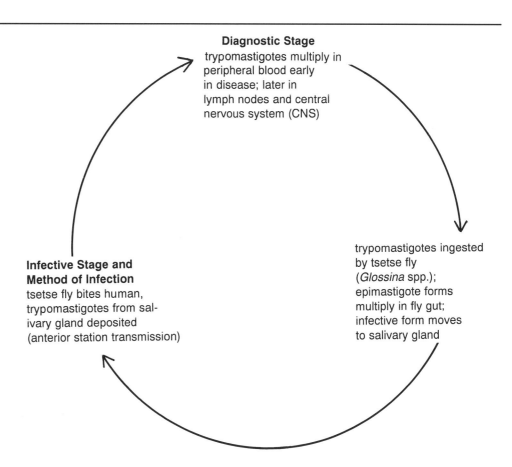

Diagnostic Stage
trypomastigotes multiply in peripheral blood early in disease; later in lymph nodes and central nervous system (CNS)

trypomastigotes ingested by tsetse fly (*Glossina* spp.); epimastigote forms multiply in fly gut; infective form moves to salivary gland

Infective Stage and Method of Infection
tsetse fly bites human, trypomastigotes from salivary gland deposited (anterior station transmission)

METHOD OF DIAGNOSIS Examine fluid from bite site chancre or buffy coat of blood for trypomastigotes during febrile period. Thick blood smears (see page 134) increase the chance of diagnosis. Multiple whole blood specimens may be needed. Thick and thin blood smears are stained with Giemsa or Wright stain. Late in infection, trypomastigotes are best found in lymph nodes or cerebrospinal fluid. Concentrating cerebrospinal fluid by centrifugation may increase the chance of recovering parasites. Animal inoculation (mice or young rats) may be helpful; trypomastigotes in patient's blood multiply in the animal.

**DIAGNOSTIC
STAGE**

Trypomastigote form in plasma

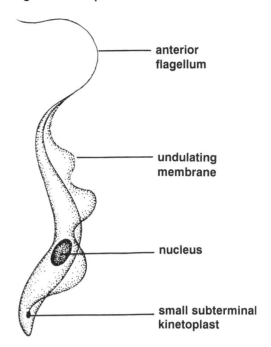

anterior
flagellum

undulating
membrane

nucleus

small subterminal
kinetoplast

15 to 30 μm x 15 to 3.5 μm

Note: Trypomastigote form
may be seen dividing
in peripheral blood.

**MAJOR
PATHOLOGY AND
SYMPTOMS**

Pathology and symptoms for both parasites include:

1. Lesion of bite site (chancre) usually seen in non-Africans.
2. Enlarged lymph nodes, especially posterior cervical chain (Winterbottom's sign).
3. Fever, headache, night sweats.
4. Joint and muscle pain.
5. Central nervous system (CNS) impairment in 6 months to 1 year with *T. b. gambiense* but in 1 month with *T. b. rhodesiense.*
6. Lethargy and motor changes.
7. Coma and death; death from cardiac failure may precede CNS symptoms in *T. b. rhodesiense.*

TREATMENT

Depends on phase of disease. Early: suramin or pentamidine; late: melarsoprol or tryparsamide, when CNS involvement has occurred.

DISTRIBUTION

Primarily Africa, East or West as noted.

OF NOTE

1. Red blood cell autoagglutination is commonly observed in vitro.
2. High levels of immunoglobulin M (IgM) and high levels of spinal fluid proteins are characteristic.
3. IgM in spinal fluid is diagnostic.

DIAGRAM 5–6
Trypanosoma cruzi
(Chagas' disease)

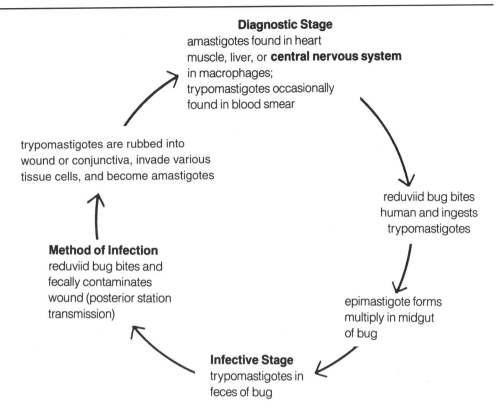

Diagnostic Stage
amastigotes found in heart
muscle, liver, or **central nervous system**
in macrophages;
trypomastigotes occasionally
found in blood smear

trypomastigotes are rubbed into
wound or conjunctiva, invade various
tissue cells, and become amastigotes

reduviid bug bites
human and ingests
trypomastigotes

Method of Infection
reduviid bug bites and
fecally contaminates
wound (posterior station
transmission)

epimastigote forms
multiply in midgut
of bug

Infective Stage
trypomastigotes in
feces of bug

METHOD OF DIAGNOSIS

1. Finding amastigotes in stained tissue scraping of skin lesion (chagoma) at bite site.
2. Identification of C-shaped trypomastigotes in blood smear during acute exacerbation.
3. **Xenodiagnosis**—allow uninfected bugs to feed on patient, then later examine bug feces for parasite.
4. Serology—Machado complement fixation test, intradermal test, or indirect hemagglutination test; endocardial, vascular, and interstitial (EVI) antibodies present.
5. L.D. bodies (amastigotes) in heart muscle postmortem.
6. Culture for epimastigotes in diphasic Novy, MacNeal, and Nicolle (NNN) medium (see page 143).

DIAGNOSTIC STAGE

Pseudocyst containing amastigote stages in heart muscle

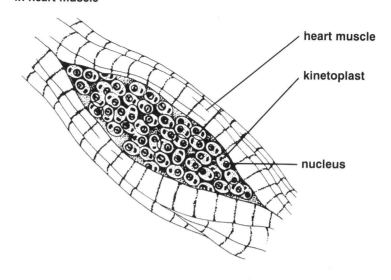

heart muscle

kinetoplast

nucleus

C- or S-shaped trypomastigote form in blood

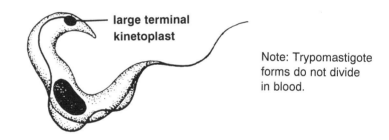

large terminal kinetoplast

Note: Trypomastigote forms do not divide in blood.

DISEASE NAMES　Chagas' disease, American trypanosomiasis

MAJOR PATHOLOGY AND SYMPTOMS

1. In chronic cases, usually in adults, there may be no history of acute illness, but enlarged, flabby heart may cause sudden death.
2. May be fever; weakness; enlarged spleen, liver, and lymph nodes.
3. Acute infection (most common in children) results in initial chagoma reaction at bite site with periorbital edema if bitten near the eye (Romaña's sign), cardiac ganglia destruction, megacolon, and often rapid death.

TREATMENT　Nifurtimox

DISTRIBUTION　Mexico, Central America, and South America; cause of 30 percent of adult deaths in Brazil. Few cases in Texas and California.

OF NOTE

1. Many animals serve as reservoir hosts in the warmer southwestern states of North America.
2. Bugs feed at night on warm-blooded hosts, frequently on the conjunctiva of the eye.
3. *T. cruzi* can cross the placenta and cause prenatal disease.

4. Autoimmune reaction by antibodies that cross-react with endocardium, vascular structures, and interstitium of smooth muscle (EVI anitbodies) may play a role in heart, colon, and esophagus dilation and atony.
5. Nonpathogenic *T. rangeli* trypomastigotes may be present in humans in Central and South America and may confuse diagnosis.

DIAGRAM 5–7
Leishmania tropica,
L. mexicana,
L. braziliensis, **and**
L. donovani **species complexes.**
(Leishmaniasis)

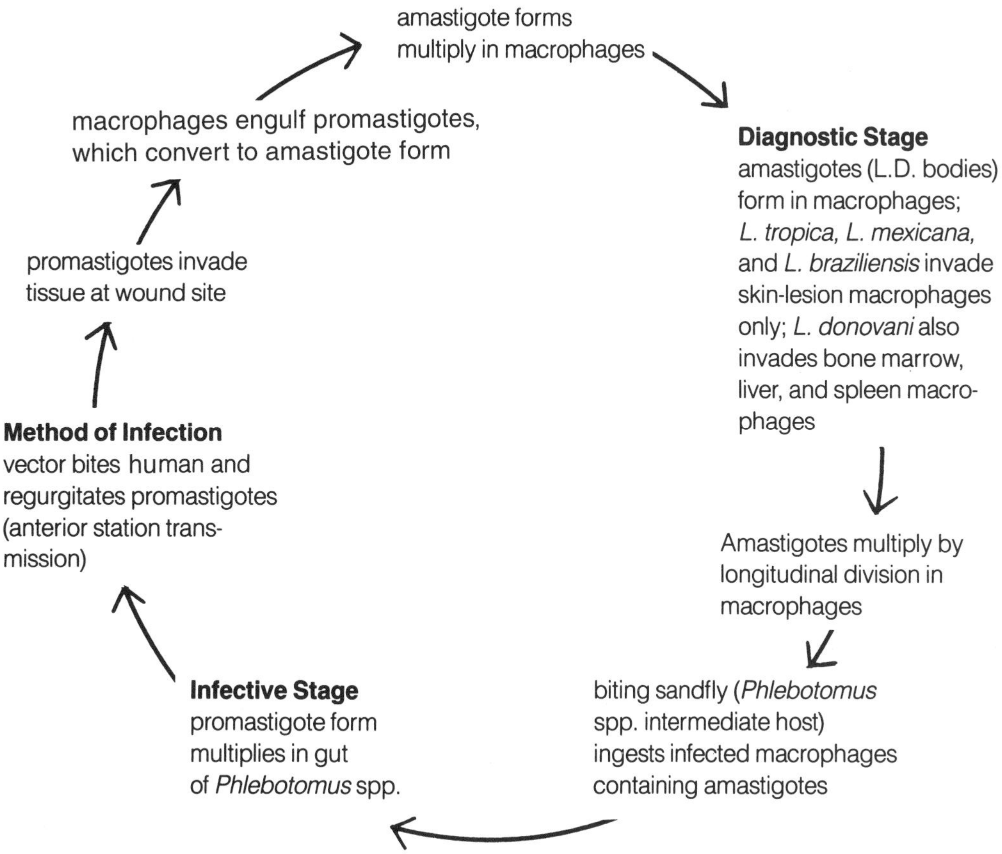

amastigote forms multiply in macrophages

macrophages engulf promastigotes, which convert to amastigote form

promastigotes invade tissue at wound site

Method of Infection
vector bites human and regurgitates promastigotes (anterior station transmission)

Infective Stage
promastigote form multiplies in gut of *Phlebotomus* spp.

Diagnostic Stage
amastigotes (L.D. bodies) form in macrophages; *L. tropica, L. mexicana,* and *L. braziliensis* invade skin-lesion macrophages only; *L. donovani* also invades bone marrow, liver, and spleen macrophages

Amastigotes multiply by longitudinal division in macrophages

biting sandfly (*Phlebotomus* spp. intermediate host) ingests infected macrophages containing amastigotes

METHOD OF DIAGNOSIS

L. tropica and *L. mexicana*—identification of amastigotes in macrophages of skin lesion.
L. braziliensis—identification of amastigotes at the periphery of the lesion.
L. donovani—identification of amastigotes in early skin lesion and L.D. bodies later in reticuloendothelial system, spleen, lymph nodes, bone marrow, and liver. Also present in feces, urine, and nasal discharges. Clinical symptoms of person in endemic area presumptive; bone marrow smears helpful; striking increase in gamma globulin; serology, skin testing, culture, and animal inoculations helpful.

SPECIMEN REQUIREMENTS

1. Fine-needle aspiration from the base of the lesion using aseptic technique is recommended. Several slides should be made and stained with Giemsa stain.
2. Cultures should be attempted for a complete diagnosis, using aspirated material and a suitable medium such as NNN.

DIAGNOSTIC STAGE

Amastigotes multiplying in tissue macrophages

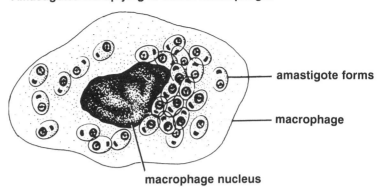

amastigote forms

macrophage

macrophage nucleus

DISEASE NAMES

L. tropica—cutaneous or Old World leishmaniasis, Oriental boil, Baghdad or Delhi boil
L. braziliensis—mucocutaneous or New World leishmaniasis, uta, espundia
L. donovani—visceral leishmaniasis, kala-azar, Dumdum fever

MAJOR PATHOLOGY AND SYMPTOMS

The type of illness is due to immunopathology in specific tissue sites.

1. *L. tropica* complex
   Incubation period: several months. One or more ulcerated, pus-filled lesions on body (indurated with macrophages); self-healing. Lesions are often moist and short-term in rural areas (infection by *L. major* lasting 3 to 6 months), dry and long-lasting in urban areas (infection by *L. tropica*, lasting 12 to 18 months).
   Treatment: (1) antimony, (2) local heat (39 to 42°C) for 12 hours on chancre

2. *L. mexicana*
   Similar to *L. tropica*. Two subspecies may cause diffuse cutaneous leishmaniasis (DCL).
   Treatment: (1) antimony, (2) amphotericin B

3. *L. braziliensis*
   Red, itchy indurated ulcer; lesions may metastasize along lymphatics; self-healing. Disfigurement of nose and ears may occur years later from chronic mucosal ulceration. Diffuse cutaneous leishmaniasis, seen mainly in Brazil, has an absence of cell-mediated immune reactivity. Note: May be caused by *L. Pifanoi*.
   Treatment: (1) antimony, (2) amphotericin B

4. *L. donovani*
   Long incubation period. Initial lesion: short-term small papules at bite site. Malarialike spiking chills and fever (double fever spike daily); sweating, diarrhea, dysentery, weight loss; splenomegaly and hepatomegaly after leishmania disseminate and multiply in visceral reticuloendothelium. Hyperplasia of tissue and organs. Progressive anemia. Causes death if untreated, often from secondary infection.
   Treatment: (1) antimony, (2) pentamidine isethionate.

DISTRIBUTION

L. tropica complex: Mediterranean area, southwestern Asia, central and northwest Africa, Central America and South America; recent cases in Texas (may be *L. mexicana*).

L. braziliensis: Central America and South America; highest concentration in Brazil and the Andes; rural disease.

L. donovani: North Africa and East Africa, Asia, Mediterranean area, and South America; primarily in young children. India and Bangladesh; primarily in adults.

OF NOTE
1. Cutaneous lesions may appear as ulcers, as cauliflowerlike masses, or as nodules.
2. Host's genetic, nutritional, and immunologic status plays a large role in pathology.
3. A variety of animals serve as reservoir hosts (e.g., gerbils and other rodents—monkeys and dogs in the New World).
4. Vaccination against *L. tropica* is common in the former U.S.S.R.
5. Leishmanian skin test becomes positive in DCL and kala-azar only after cure.
6. Elevated levels of gamma globulin are present in leishmaniasis.
7. *L. tropica* generally transmitted from humans; other parasites in the complex are primarily zoonotic.

CLASS KINETO-FRAGMINO-PHOREA

Organisms in this class are characterized by ectoplasmic cilia covering the surface, two different kinds of nuclei (a large kidney-shaped macronucleus and a small micronucleus), and other well-developed organelles such as an oral **cytostome.** Ciliates multiply asexually by binary fission and also have sexual reproduction by conjugation with exchange of micronuclei.

Balantidium coli (bal′ an-tid′ ee-um/ko′ lye) is the largest parasitic protozoon (60 μm × 40 μm) and is the only ciliate that is pathogenic for humans. *B. coli* causes dysentery in severe intestinal infections and can be found in feces in either the trophozoite or cyst state. It is probable that human infections are directly acquired through ingestion of cysts in fecally contaminated food or water.

This parasite is a tissue invader and produces intestinal lesions along the submucosa. There are also reports of vaginal infections with this organism, probably acquired by fecal contamination of the vaginal atrium.

DIAGRAM 5–8
Balantidium coli
(ciliate)

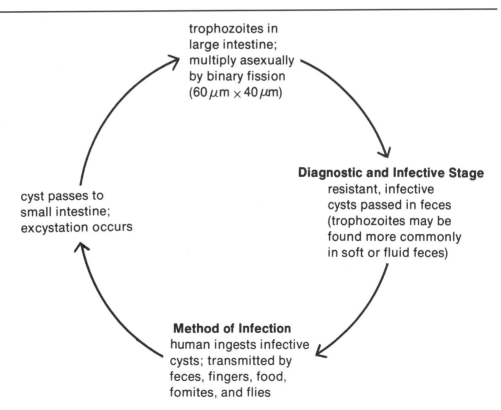

trophozoites in large intestine; multiply asexually by binary fission (60 μm × 40 μm)

Diagnostic and Infective Stage
resistant, infective cysts passed in feces (trophozoites may be found more commonly in soft or fluid feces)

Method of Infection
human ingests infective cysts; transmitted by feces, fingers, food, fomites, and flies

cyst passes to small intestine; excystation occurs

METHOD OF DIAGNOSIS Identification of trophozoites or cysts in feces or intestinal mucosa

SPECIMEN REQUIREMENTS
1. One to three stool specimens are usually sufficient. The large organisms can be noted easily under low power (100×).
2. Wet mounts of fresh or concentrated specimens are best. The organisms stain very darkly in permanently stained preparations.

DIAGNOSTIC STAGE

Cyst

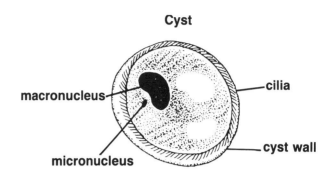

40 to 50 μm

Trophozoite

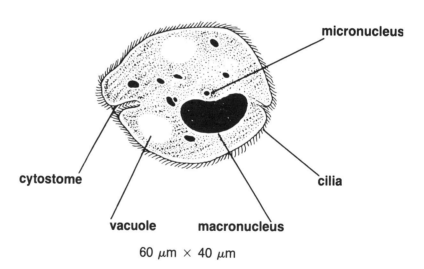

60 μm × 40 μm

DISEASE NAMES Balantidiasis, balantidial dysentery

MAJOR PATHOLOGY AND SYMPTOMS May be asymptomatic. Abdominal discomfort with mild to moderate chronic recurrent diarrhea or acute dysentery. Healthy person less likely to develop illness.

TREATMENT
1. Tetracycline
2. Iodoquinol or metronidazole

DISTRIBUTION Worldwide, especially in tropics, but rare in the United States

OF NOTE
1. Pig feces are regarded as a potential source of infection.
2. *B. coli* may invade the intestinal mucosa, causing hyperemia and hemorrhage of the bowel surface, but does not spread via bloodstream.
3. Largest protozoa and the only ciliated protozoa to infect humans.

CLASS SPOROZOA

Sporozoan parasites are obligate endoparasitic protozoa with no apparent organelles of locomotion. This class includes some of the most important and widespread parasites of humans, including those that cause malaria and toxoplasmosis (Table 5–3). Most species produce a spore form that is infective for the definitive host after it is ingested or after injection by a biting arthropod vector. All genera have a life cycle that includes both sexual (**gametocyte** production and **sporogony**) and asexual (**schizogony**) phases of reproduction. Most have a two-host life cycle.

The genus *Plasmodium* includes the sporozoon that causes human malaria. The asexual cycle (schizogony) begins when the infected female *Anopheles* mosquito (the definitive host) bites a human and injects infective **sporozoites,** which then enter cutaneous blood vessels. The sporozoites travel via blood and invade liver cells. Each becomes a **cryptozoite,** reproducing by asexual division and forming many **merozoites.** This is the exoerythrocytic cycle and is completed in 1 to 2 weeks.

The merozoites escape from the liver cells and invade circulating red blood cells (RBC). Merozoites entering RBCs become trophozoites (also known as ring forms), which then mature through the **schizont** stage in 36 to 72 hours. Each schizont produces 6 to 24 new merozoites. The timing and number of new merozoites produced differentiate the species of *Plasmodium.* When the schizont is mature, the RBC ruptures, releasing the merozoites, which in turn invade new RBCs. The cycle of RBC invasion, schizogony, and cell rupture repeats over and over again. This is the erythrocytic cycle: merozoite enters RBC→trophozoite→schizont→RBC rupture→merozoite release. Each cycle induces a **paroxysm** as toxic materials are released from the many ruptured RBCs. The paroxysm begins suddenly and is characterized by a

Table 5–3. SPOROZOANS

Order	Scientific Name	Common Name
Eucoccidiida	*Plasmodium vivax* (plaz-mo′dee-um/vye′vacks)	benign tertian malaria
Eucoccidiida	*Plasmodium falciparum* (plaz-mo′dee-um/fal-sip′uh-rum)	malignant tertian malaria
Eucoccidiida	*Plasmodium malariae* (plaz-mo′dee-um/ma-lair′ee-ee)	quartan malaria
Eucoccidiida	*Plasmodium ovale* (plaz-mo′dee-um/ovay′lee)	ovale malaria
Piroplasmida	*Babesia* spp. (bab-ee″zee′-uh)	none
Eucoccidiida	*Toxoplasma gondii* (tock″so-plaz′muh/gon′dee-eye)	toxoplasma
Eucoccidiida	*Sarcocystis* spp. (sahr″ko-sis-tis)	(*Isospora hominis* reclassified)
Eucoccidiida	*Isospora belli* (eye″sos′puh-ruh/bell-eye)	none
Uncertain	*Pneumocystis carinii* (new-moe″sis-tis/kah-reye″nee-eye)	none
Eucoccidiida	*Cryptosporidium* spp. (krip″toe-spor-i′dee-um)	none

10- to 15-minute (or longer) period of shaking chills followed by a feverish period lasting from 2 to 6 hours or more. The patient begins sweating profusely as the temperature returns to normal. The paroxysm is, in part, an allergic response to released parasitic antigens.

Later in the infection some merozoites develop into microgametocytes (male sex cells) and macrogametocytes (female sex cells). The sexual cycle (sporogony) begins when gametocytes are ingested by an *Anopheles* mosquito (definitive host) as she takes a blood meal from an infected person. The **gametes** unite in the stomach of the mosquito, forming a motile **zygote** (the **ookinete**), which then moves through and encysts on the mosquito's stomach wall. After further maturation to an **oocyst,** infective sporozoites are released from the oocyst; these migrate to the mosquito's salivary glands. The mosquito bite is now infective to the next human victim. Infective sporozoites enter via the saliva of the mosquito and travel to the liver, and the cycle begins again. Malaria can also be transmitted via blood transfusion and from contaminated needles used by drug addicts.

Drug-resistant strains of *Plasmodium* species and insecticide-resistant strains of mosquitoes, which have recently and rapidly evolved, pose major problems in controlling the disease worldwide. Control measures have essentially eliminated the disease from some countries, including the United States, but it is still a major problem in Africa, Asia, Central and South America, and areas of Europe and could be reintroduced into controlled areas.

Of the four species included in the life cycle diagram, *P. falciparum* is the most deadly; these parasites promote physiologic changes of the red cell (which develops a ''knobby'' surface) causing agglutination and lysis. Furthermore, schizogony takes place in the capillaries and blood sinuses of the brain, visceral organs, and placenta, with infected cells tending to adhere to one another and to the surrounding vessel walls. Vessels become plugged, causing local damage to the organ. Symptoms vary according to the degree of tissue anoxia and rupture of blocked capillaries. Many uninfected red cells also lyse during a paroxysm. Normal host responses to cell remnants and other parasitic debris lead to more lysis and enlargement of the spleen and liver. Other complications include renal failure caused by renal anoxia. The sudden massive intravascular lysis of RBCs, followed by hemoglobin passage in urine (blackwater fever) is related to treatment with quinine in susceptible individuals. The most severe complication, cerebral malaria, occurs when vessels in the brain become affected. Coma and death may follow.

Pathology caused by the other *Plasmodium* species is less severe, primarily because these parasites are not able to invade red cells of all ages, as are *P. falciparum* parasites. Additionally, the other species do not cause changes to the red cell membrane as seen with *P. falciparum*. Merozoites of *P. malariae* can invade only older cells, but those of *P. vivax* and *P. ovale* infect reticulocytes (immature RBCs). Inasmuch as these cell populations are small at any given time, the infection is limited by the environment provided by the host. *P. falciparum* can infect RBCs of all ages.

Plasmodium vivax is the most widely disseminated and most prevalent parasite causing malaria. There is repeated exoerythrocytic development in the liver, so that *P. vivax* can cause relapses with erythrocytic cycles starting again years after the initial infection sequence. This is thought to be due to **hypnozoites** in the liver.

DIAGRAM 5–9
Plasmodium **species
(malaria)**

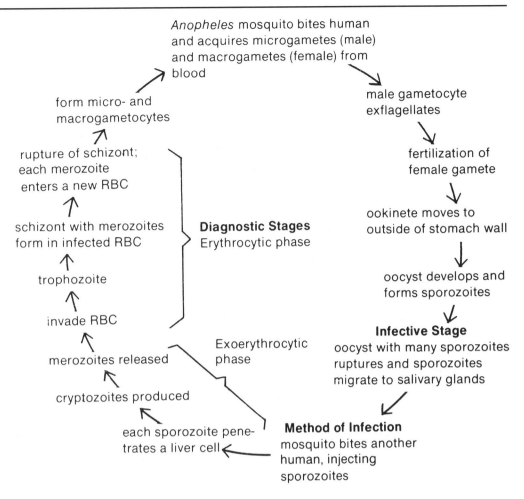

Anopheles mosquito bites human
and acquires microgametes (male)
and macrogametes (female) from
blood

form micro- and
macrogametocytes

male gametocyte
exflagellates

rupture of schizont;
each merozoite
enters a new RBC

fertilization of
female gamete

schizont with merozoites
form in infected RBC

Diagnostic Stages
Erythrocytic phase

ookinete moves to
outside of stomach wall

trophozoite

oocyst develops and
forms sporozoites

invade RBC

Infective Stage
oocyst with many sporozoites
ruptures and sporozoites
migrate to salivary glands

merozoites released

Exoerythrocytic
phase

cryptozoites produced

each sporozoite pene-
trates a liver cell

Method of Infection
mosquito bites another
human, injecting
sporozoites

**METHOD OF
DIAGNOSIS**

Demonstration and identification of trophozoites, schizonts, or gametocytes in peripheral blood. Ideally, blood should be drawn between paroxysms, as the greatest number
of parasites is likely to be present in the specimen at this time. See Disease Names, page
91, for the cycle of paroxysms for each species. Negative morning and afternoon thick-
stained smears for three consecutive days during symptoms indicate absence of infection.
Serology is helpful.

**SPECIMEN
REQUIREMENTS**

Ethylenediaminotetraacetic acid (EDTA)-preserved whole blood is preferred if antico-
agulants are used for collection, but smears should be made within 1 hour because
true stippling may not be retained (e.g., *P. vivax*).
Giemsa stain is preferred, but parasites are visible when stained with Wright stain.

**DIAGNOSTIC
STAGES**

P. falciparum

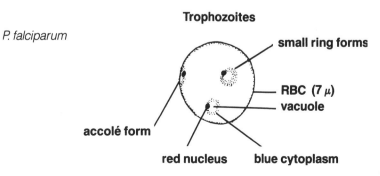

Trophozoites

small ring forms

RBC (7 μ)

vacuole

accolé form

red nucleus   **blue cytoplasm**

Continued

**Gametocyte
(crescent-shaped)**

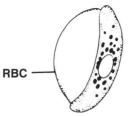

RBC

Note: Advanced trophozoites
and schizonts
generally not seen in
peripheral blood

P. malariae

**Trophozoite
(single ring)**

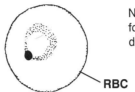

RBC

Note: Trophozoite
forms band across RBC
during early schizogony.

**Schizont
(6 to 12 merozoites)**

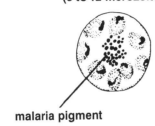

malaria pigment

**Gametocyte
(ovoid)**

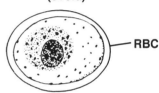

RBC

P. vivax

**Trophozoite
(single ring)**

Reticulocyte
(immature RBC 7 to 10 μ)

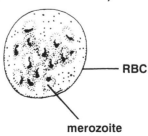

Schüffner's dots

Note: Single ring,
one-third diameter of
an RBC; invades only
immature RBCs so that
large bluish-staining cells are
parasitized.
RBC shows red-stained
Schüffner's dots, which
become visible between
15 and 20 hours following
invasion of the cell.
Note: Trophozoite is very
ameboid and assumes bizarre
shapes during early schizogony.

**Schizont
(12 to 24 merozoites)**

RBC

merozoite

**Gametocyte
(round)**

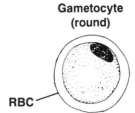

RBC

P. ovale **(rare)**	Note: Single ring, one-third diameter of RBC. RBC is oval, shows Schüffner's dots.

DISEASE NAMES

		Cyclic Paroxysms
P. falciparum	Malignant malaria	Every 36 to 48 hours
P. vivax	Tertian malaria	Every 48 hours
P. malariae	Quartan malaria	Every 72 hours
P. ovale	Ovale malaria	Every 48 hours

MAJOR PATHOLOGY AND SYMPTOMS

All cause splenic enlargement, fever and chill paroxysms, pain in the joints, and anemia from red cell destruction. Malaria pigment is deposited in tissues. *P. falciparum* infection can cause high fever, bloody urine, massive hemolysis, and brain damage from clumping of RBCs and resultant blocking of capillaries; subsequent rapid death can occur. High IgM and IgG levels suggest current or recurrent infection; elevated IgG alone indicates past infection. Quartan malaria nephropathy is immunopathologic from immune complex deposition in kidneys. *P. falciparum* infection results in massive hemolysis, hemoglobinuria (blackwater fever), and renal failure. Suspicion and response must be high for the diagnosis of malaria when a patient who has visited or lived in a malarious area shows compatible illness, because death can occur quickly if treatment is delayed.

TREATMENT

Chloroquine, quinine, pyrimethamine, sulfadiazine, tetracycline

DISTRIBUTION

P. falciparum and *P. malariae*—tropics
P. vivax—tropics, subtropics, and some temperate regions; most common species
P. ovale—West Africa
P. vivax and *P. falciparum* account for more than 95 percent of infections; primarily a rural disease; incidence significantly increasing

OF NOTE

1. *P. vivax* and *P. ovale* may cause **relapses** years later because of secondary exoerythrocytic cycles (**hypnozoites** in liver); primaquine is used to kill the liver-phase organisms of malaria.
2. *P. vivax* invades reticulocytes preferentially; therefore, counterstaining blood for reticulocytes can aid identification.
3. Inherited glucose-6-phosphate dehydrogenase deficiency and hemoglobin gene alterations (such as sickle cell inheritance) may play an evolutionary role in survival of humans in endemic areas, inasmuch as these genetic variants are incompatible with parasite survival.
4. Presence of *P. falciparum* schizonts in peripheral blood indicates very grave prognosis.
5. *P. malariae* infections may also cause a **recrudescence** or series of recrudescences for many years due to low-grade parasitemia.

BABESIA SPECIES

Ticks are the definitive hosts for the sporozoa of the *Babesia* species (subclass Piroplasmia), and occasional tick-borne human infections have been reported. In humans, the organisms multiply in red blood cells and are generally pear-shaped (2 to 4 μm), lying in pairs or tetrads. Clinical signs follow the bite of an infected tick in about 2 to 3 weeks and resemble symptoms of malaria, possibly accompanied by hemolytic anemia and mild spleen and liver disease.

Studies comparing disease symptoms found in patients in the northeastern United States with those found in patients in California indicate that more than one species of *Babesia* causes disease in humans. Cases in the Northeast are more acute and several patients have died, whereas the infections in California tend to be subclinical except in splenectomized or immunocompromised patients. *Babesia* spp. infections have been transmitted through blood transfusions.

METHOD OF DIAGNOSIS

Examination of multiple thin and thick blood smears. Parasites in red blood cells usually lie in pairs at an acute angle or as a tetrad in a Maltese cross formation. Care must be taken not to confuse *Babesia* spp. with malarial ring forms of *Plasmodium*.

DIAGNOSTIC STAGE

Babesia microti

Trophozoites

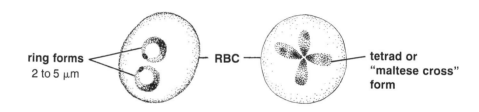

ring forms
2 to 5 μm

RBC

tetrad or
"maltese cross"
form

SPECIMEN REQUIREMENTS

Whole blood or capillary blood may be used.
Giemsa stain is preferred, but parasites are visible when stained with Wright stain.

TREATMENT

Chloroquine phosphate provides symptomatic relief but does not reduce the parasitemia.

DISTRIBUTION

Worldwide

OF NOTE

Automated differential counting instruments can lead to diagnostic problems because these machines are not designed to detect bloodborne parasites, and infections may be missed if asymptomatic.

SUBCLASS COCCIDIA

The next three genera of sporozoa to be discussed belong to the subclass **Coccidia;** schizogony occurs in a variety of nucleated cells of many species of mammals and birds, and sporogony occurs in the intestinal mucosa of the definitive host. Infective oocysts are passed in feces.

DIAGRAM 5–10
Life cycle of coccidian parasites

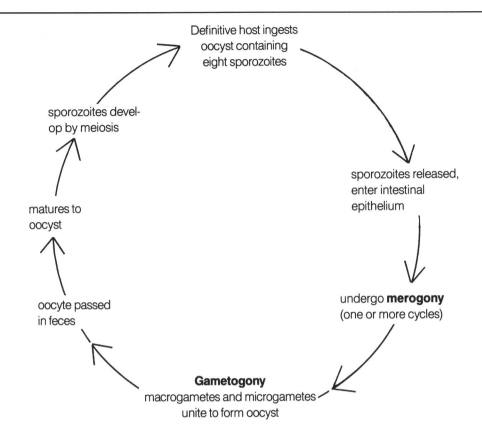

Definitive host ingests oocyst containing eight sporozoites

sporozoites develop by meiosis

matures to oocyst

oocyte passed in feces

Gametogony
macrogametes and microgametes unite to form oocyst

sporozoites released, enter intestinal epithelium

undergo **merogony** (one or more cycles)

Toxoplasma gondii *Toxoplasma gondii* is a sporozoan parasite that infects and undergoes schizogony in all nucleated cells of almost all animals and birds. The domestic cat, however, has been cited as the definitive host for this parasite, and in the cat it is an intestinal parasite, with both schizogony and sporogony occurring in the intestinal mucosa (the enteric cycle). Oocysts are shed in cat feces, and these become infective within several days for a variety of vertebrate intermediate hosts. Humans become infected by ingesting the infective oocyst in food or drink or by accidental means (e.g., from contaminated soil or cat litter). Initially, *Toxoplasma* divides mitotically in the tissues of humans as **tachyzoites,** which assume a crescentlike appearance in tissue fluids. It can also form **pseudocysts** (groups of **bradyzoites**) in brain and other tissues in which viable *Toxoplasma* organisms may remain for long periods of time, being held in check by the host's immune system.

The infection in humans is usually asymptomatic; however, it may be highly symptomatic in early infections and can mimic a variety of other infections such as infectious mononucleosis. A serious concern is that *Toxoplasma* may be transmitted across the placenta to a fetus in a mother who acquires her first infection during pregnancy. It can cause death of the fetus, mental retardation, or blindness later in life. Other sources of infection for humans, in addition to ingestion of oocysts from cat feces or from transplacental infection, are ingestion of undercooked meat containing calcified pseudocysts or milk containing **tachyzoites**. The cat becomes infected by eating infective oocysts (which are viable for up to a year in moist soil) or tissues of infected small animals. Hand-mouth transfer of oocysts from infected soil also can cause infection in humans.

TREATMENT 1. Pyrimethamine and sulfadiazine (Add folinic acid in an immunosuppressed host.)
2. Spiramycin

***Sarcocystis* spp.**   Two species of *Sarcocystis* (formerly known as *Isospora hominis*), *S. bovihominis* (cattle) and *S. suihominis* (pigs) have a life cycle similar to *Toxoplasma*. Humans, dogs, or cats can become definitive hosts if they eat uncooked beef or pork tissue containing sarcocysts. Sporozoites released from the sarcocyst invade intestinal cells and undergo gametogony, producing infective oocysts. These oocysts can be recovered in stool. Oocysts ingested by the intermediate host (cattle or pigs) release sporozoites that go to muscle tissue and form sarcocysts. Humans can also be accidental intermediate hosts. Immunocompromised humans may have severe diarrhea, fever, and weight loss when infected with this parasite. Other species of *Sarcocystis* are found in wild animal reservoir hosts.

The broadly oval oocyst contains two sporocysts each with four mature sporozoites. The sporocysts, measuring 9 to 16 μm by 8 to 12 μm, are commonly seen free in feces. Intact oocysts and individual sporozoites are rarely seen.

Isospora belli   There is one pathogenic coccidian for which the human is the definitive host, in which both schizogony and sporogony, accompanied by mild pathology, occur. This species is *Isospora belli*. Characteristic oocysts can be found in infected human feces. The oocysts of *I. belli* in a fresh fecal specimen are transparent, measuring 30 μm $\times$ 12 μm, and are immature (containing a single mass of protoplasm called the sporoblast) or, rarely, developing (containing two sporoblasts). Within 18 to 36 hours after feces are passed, each of the two sporoblasts develops a sporocyst wall and contains four sausage-shaped infective sporozoites. Full maturation takes 4 to 5 days.

This parasite is found worldwide, and transmission to humans is direct via sporulated oocysts in fecally contaminated food or water. Human infection can cause anorexia, nausea, abdominal pain, diarrhea, and possible malabsorption.

METHOD OF DIAGNOSIS
1. Oocysts are recoverable with zinc sulfate flotation technique and stain well with iodine.
2. Oocysts in polyvinyl alcohol (PVA)-preserved sediment are difficult to see because the cyst wall is very thin and refractile.
3. Although oocysts of *Sarcocystis* spp. resemble those of developed *I. belli,* they are smaller and often lose the cyst wall, and only single *Sarcocystis* sporocysts, each containing four mature sporozoites, are seen in stool samples. Oocysts of *I. belli* are undeveloped in fresh feces and retain the oocyst wall.

SPECIMEN REQUIREMENTS   Several routine fecal specimens are usually sufficient.

TREATMENT   Trimethoprim-sulfamethoxazole (TMP-SMX)

Cryptosporidium parvum   *Cryptosporidium parvum* differs from other coccidian protozoa because it forms an intracellular vacuole bounded by the host cell membrane near the outer surface of the host intestinal cell. This parasite invades the gastrointestinal mucosal surface of many vertebrate hosts, including humans. Both trophozoites and schizonts are attached to the host-cell membrane. Eight merozoites develop within the schizont and on maturation are released to begin a new schizontic cycle or to initiate a sexual cycle. Macro- and microgametocytes become mature gametes. Sexual union forms an oocyte, which then develops into an oocyst. The entire life cycle can occur within a single host, because oocysts are autoreinfective. External infection is probably acquired from food or water contaminated with oocysts from feces of animal reservoir hosts, such as calves. Human-to-human transmission occurs, and nosocomial infections have also been reported. The oocysts are immediately infective when passed in feces. The oocyst is 4 μm and contains four sporozoites.

Human infection, first reported in 1976, was thought to be infrequent and was found primarily in patients with compromised immune systems. Since then, many more cases have been reported in many populations worldwide. In 1987, an estimated 13,000 cases of gastroenteritis were reported in a 2-month period in Carroll County, Georgia, in the United States. Thirty-four percent of the patients tested were found to have *Cryptosporidium* oocysts. Follow-up studies suggested that as many as 54 percent of these cases were caused by this parasite. The source of infection was found to be the county's public water supply. This event and others indicate that infections caused by this parasite are not rare.

The symptom common to all reported cases is acute diarrhea. The disease is self-limiting in patients with normal immune systems and lasts from 1 to 2 weeks. Immuno-deficient patients, such as those with AIDS and those receiving immunosuppressant drugs, frequently develop chronic diarrhea following infection with *C. parvum*. AIDS patients have also developed respiratory cryptosporidiosis.

Cyclospora spp.

Another coccidian parasite that resembles *C. parvum* is *Cyclospora* spp. (cyanobacterium-like body [CLB]). Infection by this parasite causes a self-limiting diarrhea that may last 3 or 4 days; however, relapses often occur over a period of 2 to 3 weeks. Antidiarrheal preparations provide relief of symptoms, but no other antiparasitic therapies are available at present. Transmission of this organism, which appears primarily waterborne, can produce disease in people of all ages. It is important to differentiate this parasite from *C. parvum* and other sporozoa by careful measurement and observation of oocysts recovered in fecal specimens. Oocysts of *Cyclospora* spp. measure 8 to 10 μm and are immature, taking 5 days to develop sporozoa.

METHOD OF DIAGNOSIS

1. Oocysts are most easily recovered by flotation methods and can be observed using phase contrast (preferred) or bright field microscopy. Unstained *Cyclospora* spp. appear as glassy, wrinkled spheres.
2. Acid-fast stained smears of fecal material are also useful. Stained cells containing *Cryptosporidium* spp. appear as red spherical bodies measuring 3 to 6 μm in diameter, whereas those of *Cyclospora* spp. (8 to 10 μm in diameter) range from pink to red, and some may contain granules or have a bubbly appearance.
3. Trophozoites, schizonts, microgametocytes, and macrogametocytes of *C. parvum* can be distinguished when using the electron microscope to examine smears of biopsy material from the jejunum.

DIAGNOSTIC STAGES OF INTESTINAL COCCIDIA

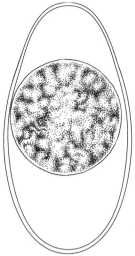

Isospora belli
immature oocyst
containing a sporoblast
15 × 30 μm

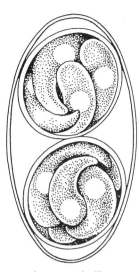

Isospora belli
mature oocyst
containing
4 sporozoites
in each sporocyst
(not seen in
fresh specimen)

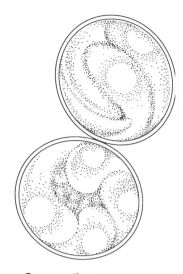

Sarcocystis spp.
2 mature sporocysts
containing 4 sporozoites each
(cyst wall gone)
9 × 12 μm (each sporocyst)

Cryptosporidium spp.
oocyst containing 4 sporozoites
4 μm

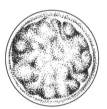

Cyclospora
immature oocyst
8 to 10 μm

Table 5–4. COCCIDIAN FORMS FOUND IN FECES

Parasite	Stage in Feces	Size	Appearance in Feces
Sarcocystis spp.	Free sporocysts	9–16 μm	Contains four sporozoites
Isospora belli	Immature oocyst	20–33 × 10–19 μm	Contains one or two immature sporoblasts
Cryptosporidium parvum	Mature oocyst	4–6 μm	Contains four sporozoites
Cyclospora spp. (CLB)	Immature oocyst	8–10 μm	Contains immature sporoblast

SPECIMEN REQUIREMENTS   Three fecal specimens collected on alternate days are usually sufficient.

TREATMENT   *I. belli*—trimethoprim-sulfamethoxazole (TMP-SMX)
C. parvum—spiramycin (experimental)
Sarcocystis spp.—none for tissue disease, antidiarrheal for accidental infection
Cyclospora spp.—none except antidiarrheal

DISTRIBUTION   Worldwide

PNEUMOCYSTIS CARINII

Pneumocystis carinii is the causative agent of atypical interstitial plasma-cell pneumonia (PCP). The classification of this parasite and its life cycle are uncertain. Both trophozoite and cyst forms exist in tissue spaces. This organism is endemic in many parts of the world and can produce pneumonia, particularly in infants, in patients with immunologic disorders such as AIDS (most common cause of death in AIDS patients), and in patients receiving immunosuppressive therapy. The organism has also been found in other tissue sites, such as lymph nodes, liver, spleen, bone marrow, and most other organs as well.

Direct-contact transmission between humans by pulmonary droplets is probable. Clinical cases of *Pneumocystis* pneumonia generally occur only in those with a predisposing debilitated state. Prognosis is poor.

METHOD OF DIAGNOSIS

1. The organism may be demonstrated intracellularly and extracellularly as cysts or trophozoites, in lung biopsies, or in lung aspirates stained with methenamine silver. The thick-walled cyst form (7 to 10 μm) contains four to eight trophozoites. The organism may appear as a single pleomorphic form (2 to 5 μm) with a double outer membrane.
2. Lung tissue assumes a honeycomb appearance.
3. Other useful stains include monoclonal immunofluorescent methods and chemofluorescent stain.

SPECIMEN REQUIREMENTS

Lung biopsy or bronchoalveolar aspirates (sputum is usually unacceptable). Sputum obtained from AIDS patients should be preserved in 10 percent formalin; it can then be processed according to the methods described.

DIAGNOSTIC STAGE

Pneumocystis carinii

Mature Cyst

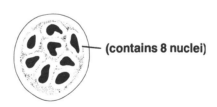

— (contains 8 nuclei)

7 to 10 μm

TREATMENT

Co-trimoxazole or pentamidine isethionate

DISTRIBUTION

Worldwide

OF NOTE

Recent evidence suggests that *P. carinii* may actually be a fungus, but to date it is still considered a Protozoa.

MICRO-SPORIDIA

The microsporidia have recently been recognized as tissue parasites in immunocompromised patients. In humans, they are small (1 to 2.5 μm), obligate intracellular parasites that can inhabit all body tissues. They consist of four named genera and one "catch-all" genus (*Microsporidium* spp.), which is currently used for species that have not yet been fully described. The other genera are *Enterocytozoon* spp., *Encephalitozoon* spp., *Nosema* spp., and *Pleistophora* spp. These organisms inject infective contents from the spore into the host cell through a small tube. The organism continues to multiply inside the host cell by binary fission (merogony) or multiple fission (schizogony) and sexual reproduction (sporogony). Merogony and sporogony may happen at the same time in the same cell. Spores are produced with thick walls and, for *Enterocytozoon bieneusi*, are released into the intestine and passed in stool. Other hosts become infected by ingesting spores. Microsporidia have been found in the CNS, eyes, lungs, kidney, myocardium, liver, and adrenal cortex and have been found associated with other diseases, such as leprosy, tuberculosis, schistosomiasis, malaria, and Chagas' disease. Infection by *Enterocytozoon bieneusi* is the most frequent microsporidial infection found in AIDS patients.

METHOD OF DIAGNOSIS
1. Diagnosis is accomplished by histology using acid-fast and periodic acid–Schiff (PAS) stains or electron microscopy.
2. Very thin acid-fast or trichrome-stained fecal smears may reveal spores. Positive controls are necessary.

SPECIMEN REQUIREMENTS
1. Tissue biopsy materials for processing in histology. (Best staining with PAS, methenamine silver, or acid-fast stains.)
2. Three fecal collections on alternate days. Thin smears are necessary.

TREATMENT No satisfactory treatment is currently available.

DISTRIBUTION Worldwide

OF NOTE Double infections with Cryptosporidia and Microsporidia are common.

Table 5–5 reviews the life cycles and other important information about the Protozoa. Study these carefully before taking the chapter post-test.
Consult Color Plates 72 to 126.

Table 5–5. PATHOGENIC PROTOZOA

Scientific and Common Name	Epidemiology	Disease-Producing Form and Its Location in Hosts	How Infection Occurs	Major Disease Manifestations, Diagnostic Stage, and Specimen of Choice
Entamoeba histolytica (amebic dysentery)	Worldwide	Trophozoites in large intestinal mucosa, liver, or other tissues	Ingestion of cyst in fecally contaminated food or water	Enteritis with abdominal pain and bloody dysentery Diagnosis: cysts and trophozoites in feces
Blastocystis hominis (None)	Worldwide	Protozoa in intestine	Ingestion of organisms in fecally contaminated food or water	Diarrhea, fever, abdominal pain, vomiting
Acanthamoeba spp. (chronic meningoencephalitis)	Worldwide	Trophozoites and cysts in tissues of brain, eye, skin, etc.	Accidental entrance through skin lesion	Slow disease development (over 10 days)
Naegleria fowleri (primary amebic meningoencephalitis)	Worldwide	Amebic trophozoites in brain	Accidental entrance of free-living water-borne trophozoites through nasopharynx mucosa	Rapid death

Table 5–5. PATHOGENIC PROTOZOA (Continued)

Scientific and Common Name	Epidemiology	Disease-Producing Form and Its Location in Hosts	How Infection Occurs	Major Disease Manifestations, Diagnostic Stage, and Specimen of Choice
Dientamoeba fragilis (none)	Worldwide	Trophozoites in large intestine	Ingestion of trophozoite (?)	Diarrhea Diagnosis: trophozoites in feces (no cysts formed)
Giardia lamblia (traveler's diarrhea)	Worldwide	Trophozoites in large intestinal mucosa	Ingestion of cysts in fecally contaminated food or water	Mild to severe dysentery; malabsorption syndrome Diagnosis: cysts and trophozoites in feces
Trichomonas vaginalis (trich)	Worldwide	Trophozoites in urethra or vagina	Sexual contact	Irritating, frothy vaginal discharge in women; men usually asymptomatic Diagnosis: trophozoites in urine or vaginal smear (no cysts formed)
Leishmania tropica complex (Oriental boil)	Mediterranean area, Asia, Africa, Central America	Amastigotes in macrophages of skin lesion	Bite of *Phlebotomus* spp. (sandfly)	Self-healing skin lesion Diagnosis: amastigotes in macrophages around lesion
Leishmania mexicana complex (New World cutaneous leishmaniasis)	Mexico, Central and South America	Amastigotes in macrophages of skin lesions	Bite of *Lutzomyia* spp.	Self-healing skin lesion; some species cause diffuse cutaneous leishmaniasis
Leishmania braziliensis complex (New World leishmaniasis, espundia)	Central and South America, especially Brazil	Amastigotes in macrophages of skin lesion and mucocutaneous tissue	Bite of *Lutzomyia* spp. and *Psychodopygus* spp.	Self-healing skin lesion, later ulceration of cephalic mucocutaneous tissue Diagnosis: recovery of amastigotes from lesion
Leishmania donovani (kala-azar)	Mediterranean area, Asia, Africa, South America	Amastigotes in macrophages in skin lesion and somatic organs	Bite of *Phlebotomus* spp.	Initial skin lesion, later daily double-spiking fever, enlarged liver and spleen, death in late stages Diagnosis: L.D. bodies in early lesion, organ tissue biopsy later
Trypanosoma brucei gambiense (sleeping sickness)	West Africa	Trypomastigote in blood, lymph nodes, later in CNS	Bite of *Glossina* spp. (tsetse fly)	Fever, lymphadenopathy (Winterbottom's sign), enlarged spleen and liver, lethargy, and death Diagnosis: trypomastigotes in blood smear, CSF
Trypanosoma brucei rhodesiense (sleeping sickness)	East Africa	Trypomastigote in blood, lymph nodes, later in CNS	Bite of *Glossina* spp. (tsetse fly)	Fever, lymphadenopathy (Winterbottom's sign), enlarged spleen and liver, lethargy, and death Course more acute and fatal than *T. gambiense* Diagnosis: trypomastigotes in blood smear

Table continued on following page

Table 5–5. PATHOGENIC PROTOZOA (Continued)

Scientific and Common Name	Epidemiology	Disease-Producing Form and Its Location in Hosts	How Infection Occurs	Major Disease Manifestations, Diagnostic Stage, and Specimen of Choice
Trypanosoma cruzi (Chagas' disease)	South America	C-shaped trypomastigote and epimastigote forms early in blood; later, L.D. bodies in heart and other tissues	Infected feces of *Triatoma* spp. (kissing bug) rubbed into bite site	Fever, enlarged spleen and liver, Romaña's sign (edema around eyes), chronic damage to heart and alimentary tract. Acute death, especially in children. Diagnosis: trypomastigotes in blood; xenodiagnosis
Balantidium coli (balantidial dysentery)	Worldwide	Trophozites in large intestinal mucosa	Ingestion of cysts in fecally contaminated food or water	Moderate or mild dysentery. Diagnosis: trophozoites or cysts in feces
Plasmodium vivax (benign tertian malaria)	Tropics, subtropics, some temperate regions	Schizogony and gametocytes in RBCs	*Anopheles* spp. mosquito transmits sporozoites	Cyclic fever, chills, enlarged spleen, parasites in red blood cells. Diagnosis: malarial forms in blood smear
Plasmodium malariae (quartan malaria)	Tropics	Schizogony and gametocytes in RBCs	*Anopheles* spp. mosquito transmits sporozoites	Cyclic fever, chills, enlarged spleen, parasites in RBCs; relapses. Diagnosis: malarial forms in blood smear
Plasmodium falciparum (malignant malaria)	Tropics	Trophozoites and gametocytes in peripheral RBCs	*Anopheles* spp. mosquito transmits sporozoites	Cyclic fever, chills, enlarged spleen, parasites in RBCs. Blackwater fever from hemoglobin in urine, blockage of capillaries, death. Diagnosis: malarial forms in blood smear
Plasmodium ovale (ovale malaria)	West Africa	Schizogony and gameto cytes in RBCs	*Anopheles* spp. mosquito transmits sporozoites	Cyclic fever, chills, enlarged spleen, parasites in RBCs. Diagnosis: malarial forms in blood smear
Toxoplasma gondii (toxoplasmosis)	Worldwide	Trophozoites intracellularly in all organs; pseudocysts in brain and other tissue	Ingestion of oocysts; ingestion of trophozoites or pseudocysts in undercooked meat; congenital passage of trophozoites	Fever, enlarged lymph nodes. In fetus or neonate: damage or death. Can cause acute infection in immunosuppressed patient. Diagnosis: serology
Isospora belli (none)	Worldwide	Schizogony and gametogony stages in intestinal epithelium	Ingestion of infective oocysts	Diarrhea. Diagnosis: oocyst and sporocysts in feces

Table 5–5. PATHOGENIC PROTOZOA (Continued)

Scientific and Common Name	Epidemiology	Disease-Producing Form and Its Location in Hosts	How Infection Occurs	Major Disease Manifestations, Diagnostic Stage, and Specimen of Choice
Sarcocystis spp. (none) (*zoonosis*)	Worldwide	Sarcocyst in muscle Oocyst formation in intestine	Ingestion of sarcocyst from undercooked meat or oocyst from water or food contaminated by infected cattle or pigs	Sarcocysts (Miescher's tubes) in muscle do not generally cause problems Diagnosis: tissue biopsy; oocysts in feces
Pneumocystis carinii (none)	Europe, Asia, United States	Cysts in lungs	Unknown	Interstitial plasma cell pneumonia in immunosuppressed patients. Frequently seen in AIDS patients. Diagnosis: cysts or pleomorphic forms in bronchoalveolar lavage or transbronchial biopsy. Honeycomb appearance of lung tissue.
Cryptosporidium spp. (none)	Worldwide	Invades GI tract mucosa	Probably by ingestion of fecally contaminated food or water; human-to-human transmission	Diarrhea Diagnosis: trophozoites and schizonts in biopsy of jejunum
Babesia spp. (*B. microti* in the United States) (none) (*zoonosis*)	Worldwide	*Babesia* trophozoites in RBCs	Tick bite (*Ixodes scapularis*); rarely, via blood transfusion	Fever; symptoms can resemble malaria Diagnosis: trophozoites in blood smear

You have now completed the material on Protozoa. After reviewing this material with the aid of your learning objectives, proceed to the post-test.

BIBLIOGRAPHY   **Intestinal Protozoa**

Arean, VM, and Koppisch, E: Balantidiosis: A review and report cases. Am J Pathol 32:1089, 1956.

Babb, RR, Peck, OC, and Vescia, FG: Giardiasis: A cause of traveler's diarrhea. JAMA 217:1359, 1971.

Brandborg, LL, Goldberg, SB, and Briedenboch, WC: Human coccidiosis—A possible cause of malabsorption. The life cycle in small bowel mucosal biopsies as a diagnostic feature. N Engl J Med 283:1306, 1970.

Mahmoud, AAF, and Warren, KS: Algorithms in the diagnosis and management of exotic diseases. II. Giardiasis. J Infect Dis 131:621, 1975.

Martinez-Palomo, A (ed): Amebiasis. In *Human Parasitic Diseases,* Vol 2. Elsevier, New York, 1986.

Meyer, EA (ed): Giardiasis. In *Human Parasitic Diseases,* Vol 3. Elsevier, New York, 1990.

Pritchard, JH, et al: Diagnosis of focal hepatic lesions. Combined radioisotope and ultrasound techniques. JAMA 229:1463, 1974.

Spice, WM, Cruz-Rayes, JA, and Achers, JP: Molecular and cell biology of opportunistic infections in AIDS. *Entamoeba histolytica.* Mol Cell Biol Hum Dis Ser 2:95–137, 1993.

Thompson, RCA, Reynoldson, JA, and Mendis, AHW: *Giardia* and giardiasis. Adv Parasitol 32:72–160, 1993.

Zierdt, CH: Blastocystis hominis—past and future. Clin Microbiol Rev 4:61-79, 1991.

Atrial and Blood Protozoa

Atias, A, et al: Mega-esophagus, megacolon and Chagas' disease in Chile. Gastroenterology 44:433, 1963.

Avila, JC, and Harris, JR (eds): *Subcellular Biochemistry,* Vol 18, Intracellular Parasites. Plenum Press, New York, 1992.

Berger, BJ, and Fairlamb, AH: Interactions between immunity and chemotherapy in the treatment of trypanosomiasis and leishmaniasis. Parasitology 105 (suppl):71–78, 1992.

Brown, MT: Trichomoniasis. Practitioner 207:639, 1972.

Chang, KP, and Bray, RS (eds): Leishmaniasis. In *Human Parasitic Diseases,* Vol 1. Elsevier, New York, 1985.

Cohen, S: Immunity to malaria. Proc R Soc Lond B Biol Sci 203:323, 1979.

Convit, J, Pinardi, ME, and Rondon, AJ: Diffuse cutaneous leishmaniasis: A disease due to an immunologic defect of the host. Trans R Soc Trop Med Hyg 66:603, 1972.

Cossio, PM, et al: Chagasic cardiopathy. Demonstration of a serum gamma globulin factor which reacts with endocardium and vascular structures. Circulation 49:13, 1974.

Dye, C, Vidor, E, and Dereure, J: Serological diagnosis of leishmaniasis on detecting infection as well as disease. Epidemiol Infect 110(3): 647–656, 1993.

Eling, WM, et al: The need for live parasites for long-term immunity in malaria. Acta Leidensia 60(1):167–175, 1991.

Garnham, PCC: *Malaria Parasites and Other Haemosporidia.* Blackwell Scientific Publications, Oxford, 1966.

Goodwin, LG: The pathology of African trypanosomiasis. Trans R Soc Trop Med Hyg 65:797, 1970.

Grunwaldt, R.: Babesiosis on Shelter Island. NY State Journal of Medicine 77:1320, 1977.

Hubsch, RM, Sulzer, AJ, and Kagan, IG: Evaluation of an autoimmune-type antibody in the sera of patients with Chagas' disease. J Parasitol 62:523, 1976.

Kaushik, A, et al: Malarial placental infection and low birth weight babies. J Commun Dis 24(2):65–69, 1992.

Luzzatto, L, Usanga, EA, and Reddy, S: Glucose-6 phosphate dehydrogenase deficient red cells: Resistance to infection with malarial parasites. Science 164:839, 1969.

Mahmoud, AAF, and Warren, KS: Algorithms in the diagnosis and management of exotic diseases, IV. American trypanosomiasis. J Infect Dis 132:121, 1975.

Miller, LH, et al: Erythrocyte receptors for *(Plasmodium knowlesi)* malaria: Duffy blood group determinants. Science 189:561, 1975.

Pepin, J, and Milord, F: The treatment of human African trypanosomiasis. Adv Parasitol 33:2–47, 1994.

Szarfman, A, et al: Investigation of the EVI antibody in parasitic diseases other than American trypanosomiasis. An anti-skeletal muscle antibody in leishmaniasis. Am J Trop Med Hyg 24:19, 1975.

Targett, GA: Virulence and the immune response in malaria. Mem Inst Oswaldo Cruz 87 (suppl) 5:127–144, 1992.

White, NJ, and HO, M: The pathophysiology of malaria. Adv Parasitol 31:84–173, 1992.

Other Protozoa

Aspock, H, and Pollak, A: Prevention of prenatal toxoplasmosis by serological screening of pregnant women in Austria. Scand J Infect Dis Suppl 84:32–37, 1992.

Babb, RR, Differding, JT, and Trollope, ML: Cryptosporidia enteritis in a healthy professional athlete. Am J Gastroenterol 77:833–834.

Baselski, VS, et al: Rapid detection of *Pneumocystis carinii* in bronchoalveolar lavage samples by using Cellufluor staining. J Clin Microbiol 28:393–394, 1990.

Bryan, RT, and Wilson, M: Clinical Casebook: Toxoplasmosis. Laboratory Management 26(8):40, 1988.

Bunyarartvej, S, Bunyawongwiroj, P, and Nitiyanant, P: Human intestinal sarcosporidiosis: Report of six cases. Am J Trop Med Hyg 31:36–41, 1982.

Camargo, ME, et al: Immunoglobulin G and immunoglobulin M enzyme-linked immunosorbent assays and defined toxoplasmosis serological patterns. Infect Immun 21:55, 1978.

Carter, RF: Primary amoebic meningoencephalitis. An appraisal of present knowledge. Trans R Soc Trop Med Hyg 66:193, 1972.

Centers for Disease Control: Primary amebic meningoencephalitis: California, Florida, New York. Morbidity Mortality Weekly Report 27:343, 1978.

Current, WL, and Barcia, LS: Cryptosporidiosis. Clin Microbiol Rev 4:325–358, 1991.

Cursons, RT, Brown, TJ, and Keyes, EA: Virulence of pathogenic free-living amebae. J Parasitol 64:744, 1978.

Cushion, MT, and Ebbets, D: Growth and metabolism of *Pneumocystis carinii* in axenic culture. J Clin Microbiol 28:1385–1394, 1990.

Edman, JC, et al: Ribosomal RNA sequence shows *Pneumocystis carinii* to be a member of the fungi. Nature 334:519–522, 1988.

Egger, MD, et al: Symptoms and transmission of intestinal cryptosporidiosis. Arch Dis Child 65:445–447, 1990.

Frenkel, JL: Toxoplasmosis and pneumocytosis: Clinical and laboratory aspects in immunocompetent and compromised hosts. In Prier, JE and Friedman, H (eds): *Opportunistic Pathogens.* University Park Press, Baltimore, 1974, pp 203–259.

Garcia, LS: Intestinal coccidia and microsporidia in non-AIDS patients. Clinical Microbiology Newsletter 11:169–172, 1989.

Greaves, T, and Strigle, S: The recognition of *Pneumocystis carinii* in routine Papanicolaou stained smears. Acta Cytol 29:714–720, 1985.

Hollister, WS, Canning, EV, Wilcox, A: Evidence for widespread occurrence of antibodies to *Encephalitozoon cuniculi* (microspora) in man provided by ELISA and other serological tests. Parasitology 102:33–45, 1991.

Jackson, MH, and Hutchison, WM: The prevalence and source of *Toxoplasma* infection in the environment. Adv Parasitol 28:55–105, 1989.

Kim, HK, and Hughes, WT: Comparison of methods for the identification of *Pneumocystis carinii* in pulmonary aspirates. Am J Clin Pathol 60:462, 1973.

Kim, YK, et al: Evaluation of calcofluor white stain for detection of *Pneumocystis carinii.* Diagn Microbiol Infect Dis 13:307–310, 1990.

Kinnig, P, Piekarski, G, Heydorn, AO: Sarcosporidiosis *(Sarcocystis suihominis)* in man. Immunol Infect 7:170–177, 1979.

Long, EG, et al: Morphologic and staining characteristics of a cyanobacterium-like organism associated with diarrhea. J Infect Dis 164:199–202, 1991.

Markus, MB: *Sarcocystis* and sarcocystosis in domestic animals and man. Adv Vet Sci Comp Med 22:159, 1978.

Metcalf, TW, et al: Microsporidial keratoconjunctivitis in a patient with AIDS. Br J Ophthalmol 76:177–178, 1992.

Moore, JA, and Frankel, JA: Respiratory and enteric cryptosporidiosis in humans. Arch Pathol Lab Med 115:1160–1162, 1991.

Murray, J, et al: Pulmonary complications of the acquired immunodeficiency syndrome: Report of a National Heart, Lung and Blood Institute workshop. N Engl J Med 310:1682–1688, 1984.

National Cancer Institute: *Monograph No. 43. Symposium on Pneumocytis Carinii Infection.* US Dept of Health, Education, and Welfare, National Institutes of Health, Bethesda, 1976.

Orenstein, JM: Microsporidiosis in the acquired immunodeficiency syndrome. J Parasitol 77:843–864, 1991.

Pitchenik, A, et al: Sputum examination for the diagnosis of *Pneumocystis carinii* pneumonia in the acquired immunodeficiency syndrome. Am Rev Respir Dis 133:226–229, 1986.

Stover, DE, et al: Bronchoalveolar lavage in the diagnosis of diffuse pulmonary infiltrates in the immunosuppressed host. Ann Intern Med 101:1–7, 1984.

Tzipori, S: Cryptosporidiosis in perspective. Adv Parasitol 27:63–129, 1988.

Wakefield, AE, et al: *Pneumocystis carinii* shows DNA homology with the ustomycetous red yeast fungi. Mol Microbiol 6:1903–1911, 1992.

Webber, R, et al: Improved light-microscopical detection of microsporidia spores in stool and duodenal aspirates. N Engl J Med 326:161–166, 1992.

Zoonoses

Coatney, GR: The simian malarias: Zoonosis, anthroponosis or both? Am J Trop Med Hyg 20:795, 1971.

Levine, ND: Protozoan parasites of nonhuman primates as zoonotic agents. Laboratory Animal Care 20:371, 1970.

POST-TEST

1. Matching: select the one best answer: **(36 points)**

   a. _____ malaria parasite with 6 to 12 merozoites in the schizont

   b. _____ C- or U-shaped body with a large kinetoplast

   c. _____ large kidney-shaped nucleus

   d. _____ trophozoite ingests red blood cells

   e. _____ large glycogen vacuole

   f. _____ schizonts not seen in peripheral blood

   g. _____ pseudocysts in brain

   h. _____ nonpathogenic

   i. _____ oocysts found in human feces

   j. _____ commonly causes relapses of malaria

   k. _____ transmitted by tsetse fly

   l. _____ pathogenic intestinal flagellate

   1. *Isospora belli*
   2. *Toxoplasma gondii*
   3. *Plasmodium vivax*
   4. *Plasmodium malariae*
   5. *Plasmodium falciparum*
   6. *Trypanosoma brucei gambiense*
   7. *Trypanosoma cruzi*
   8. *Entamoeba histolytica*
   9. *Entamoeba hartmanni*
   10. *Endolimax nana*
   11. *Iodamoeba bütschlii*
   12. *Giardia lamblia*
   13. *Trichomonas vaginalis*
   14. *Balantidium coli*

2. How would you differentiate *Entamoeba histolytica* from *Entamoeba coli* in a fecal smear? **(9 points)**

3. Define: **(20 points)**
   a. trophozoite
   b. cyst
   c. sporozoite
   d. schizogony
   e. carrier
   f. oocyst
   g. pseudocyst
   h. L.D. body
   i. paroxysm
   j. atrium

4. State method of infection for each of the following diseases: **(20 points)**
   a. kala-azar
   b. giardiasis
   c. Chagas' disease
   d. toxoplasmosis
   e. trichomonal urethritis
   f. balantidial dysentery
   g. babesiosis
   h. malaria
   i. sleeping sickness
   j. cutaneous leishmaniasis

5. Draw the ring form(s) in a red blood cell for each of the following: **(15 points)**
   a. *Plasmodium vivax*   b. *Plasmodium malariae*   c. *Plasmodium falciparum*

Each of the following multiple choice questions is worth **2 points.**

6. Charcot-Leyden crystals may be noted when examining fecal preparations. These crystals are associated with the immune response, and are thought to be breakdown products of:
   a. eosinophils
   b. lymphocytes
   c. macrophages
   d. monocytes
   e. neutrophils

7. The two parasitic organisms most commonly associated with waterborne outbreaks of diarrhea include:
   a. *Blastocystis hominis* and *Isospora belli*
   b. *Entamoeba coli* and *Giardia lamblia*

Continued

   c. *Entamoeba histolytica* and *Endolimax nana*

   d. *Giardia lamblia* and *Cryptosporidium parvum*

   e. *Trichomonas hominis* and *Toxoplasma gondii*

8. The malaria parasite characterized by the presence of multiple ring forms or "banana" gametocytes in RBCs is:

   a. *Babesia* spp.

   b. *Plasmodium falciparum*

   c. *Plasmodium malariae*

   d. *Plasmodium ovale*

   e. *Plasmodium vivax*

9. The characteristic that most clearly differentiates cysts of *Iodamoeba bütschlii* from other amebic cysts is/are:

   a. chromatoid bars with rounded ends

   b. eight nuclei with eccentrically located karyosomes

   c. ingested bacteria and RBCs

   d. a large glycogen vacuole

   e. a vacuolated cytoplasm

10. Motile amebae measuring 10 μm are noted when examining a wet mount of spinal fluid. The amoeba most likely is:

   a. *Acanthamoeba* spp.

   b. *Dientamoeba fragilis*

   c. *Entamoeba histolytica*

   d. *Iodamoeba bütschlii*

   e. *Naegleria fowleri*

11. A blood parasite that invades reticulocytes, is characterized by single ring forms and Schüffner's dots, and may cause a true relapse is:

   a. *Babesia* spp.

   b. *Plasmodium falciparum*

   c. *Plasmodium malariae*

   d. *Plasmodium ovale*

   e. *Plasmodium vivax*

CHAPTER 6

Arthropoda

LEARNING OBJECTIVES

Upon completion of this chapter, the student will be able to:

1 State the criteria used for taxonomic classification of the **Arthropoda.**
2 State the general description of each order of Arthropoda that contains genera of medical importance.
3 State the definitions of terminology specific for Arthropoda.
4 State the definitions of complete and incomplete metamorphosis and give examples of each.
5 Identify Arthropoda to class by morphologic criteria.
6 Differentiate between Acarina and Insecta.
7 Describe the type of life cycle for each Arthropoda class.
8 Contrast the role of Arthropoda as intermediate hosts rather than as transport hosts for various parasites and microorganisms.
9 Identify the specific genus of Arthropoda serving as the required intermediate host for various helminth and protozoal infections.
10 Given an illustration or photograph (or actual specimen, with sufficient laboratory experience), identify diagnosic stages of Arthropoda.
11 Discuss problems caused by the Arthropoda that have an impact on humans, and propose solutions for these problems.
12 Propose method(s) of prevention of infestation caused by arthropods.
13 Propose methods of control of Arthropoda, based upon life cycles.

The phylum Arthropoda includes the segmented invertebrates that have a protective **chitinous exoskeleton** and bilaterally paired jointed appendages. The head has structures adapted for sensory and chewing or piercing functions. Eyes are single or compound. Digestive, respiratory, excretory, and nervous systems are present. The body cavity (the hemocele) is an open space filled with a bloodlike substance.

This large group is divided into five classes, and three of these **(Insecta, Arachnida, and Crustacea)** contain most of the medically important arthropods. The important disease-producing genera listed in Table 6–1 (page 116) are members of various families. The Arthropoda is the largest phylum, containing over 80 percent of all animal life. It also directly causes or transmits more than 80 percent of all diseases. It is of major economic importance to agriculture, with both beneficial and destructive effects.

All Arachnida and most Insecta develop from egg to adult by a process called **metamorphosis.** Incomplete or hemimetabolous metamorphosis has three stages: (1) egg, (2) **nymph,** and (3) **imago,** the sexually mature adult. The nymph, a miniature adult, molts several times before it becomes an adult. The nymphal form after each molt is called an **instar.** Wings of flying insects increase in size with each instar. Lice, bugs, and arachnids are hemimetabolous.

Complete or holometabolous metamorphosis has four stages: (1) egg, (2) larva, (3) **pupa,** and (4) imago. Insect larvae appear as segmented wormlike organisms and mature through a series of instars that finally enclose themselves inside a case or pupa. After a time, the transformed imago emerges. Flies, mosquitoes, and fleas are holometabolous.

Development of most crustaceans is by incomplete metamorphosis; however, the names of the stages are different. Eggs hatch, releasing free-swimming **nauplius** larvae that molt several times to become mature adults. Some species, however, undergo complete metamorphosis; the nauplius develops into a **cypris** larva (a stage similar to the pupa), and the transformed larva emerges as an adult.

It is crucial that you understand the importance of the Arthropoda—both as parasites themselves and as vectors of other disease-causing microorganisms. Although some insects are parasites of humans (e.g., ectoparasites such as lice, mosquitoes, and ticks that feed on blood), other insects play an important role as vectors that transmit a variety of diseases. Elimination of the vector is a frequently attempted method of parasite control. Therefore, it is important to know which insect species comprise an integral part of a parasite's life cycle and also to understand the life cycle of the insect itself in order to initiate proper measures of control.

Mechanical transfer of infective organisms from feces or contaminated soil to food or utensils by the feet or mouth parts of insects, coupled with inadequate protection of food and inadequate personal hygiene, provides the means by which a person may contract an infection. Mechanical transfer implies that no further development or growth of the parasite occurs in the insect, even if the parasite is carried inside the insect and released in the insect's feces or is injected into the host by the biting insect. A biologic vector, by contrast, requires that growth and development of the parasite occur inside the insect. Insects may serve as either definitive or intermediate hosts. The infective parasites that develop in the insect either are injected directly into a new host or, in a few species, are deposited on the host's skin.

Some pathogens can be passed from an adult insect to its offspring if the organism penetrates the egg(s) in vivo. This is known as transovarial transmission. If the pathogen is able to survive in each part of the cycle (egg→nymph→adult), it has been transmitted trans-stadially. The term vertical transmission is used to describe these phenomena and means that parasites are passed from generation to generation within the same species. Certain diseases are maintained by tick vectors via vertical transmission. For example, the tick *Ixodes scapularis* is the vector for *Babesia* spp. Merogony occurs inside the tick, and some of the merozoites invade tick eggs, causing the next generation to be infected.

Besides mechanical or biologic disease transmission, other major problems caused by insects are annoyance, delayed or immediate hypersensitivity reactions to bites (including fatal anaphylaxis), blood loss, secondary bacterial infections in open insect bite sites, injection of toxins or venoms, loss of food crops, loss of animal productivity, and **myiasis.**

Myiasis is caused by larvae of non-blood-sucking flies invading tissue. Eggs or larvae may be deposited directly on skin or are transferred to the body from contaminated soil. The larvae of some fly species, however, must live in living tissue. This type of myiasis is called obligate myiasis. Although myiasis is more commonly seen in animals, humans may serve as host for several species. For example, the fly *Cochliomyia hominovorax* causes the disease known as primary screwworm. The fly is attracted to open wounds or nasal drainage, where it deposits its eggs. Larvae hatch in 11 to 22 hours, invade the skin, and begin feeding on tissue. Symptoms depend on the site of invasion, but pain, swelling, and subcutaneous larval migration occur in most cases. Many other fly larvae cause similar problems worldwide, especially in children and livestock herders. Facultative myiasis occurs when larvae enter living tissue after feeding on decaying tissue such as that found in neglected wounds. The larvae need decaying tissue for food, and the myiasis in living tissue is only passive. Many filth flies are attracted to wounded, dead, or decaying animals. This myiasis has been reported in elderly, immobile patients with open wounds. Larvae have been recovered from the ear, the nose, and even from the urogenital tract. Accidental ingestion of fly eggs or larvae may produce intestinal myiasis, resulting in various gastrointestinal symptoms.

Mechanical trauma is caused by a variety of insects including bees, wasps, ants, spiders, scorpions, centipedes, and millipedes. Some people suffer severe allergic reactions to bee and spider venoms. Bee toxins are similar to viperine snake venom in having a hemolyzing factor, but they also contain histamine. Allergic individuals may exhibit symptoms of anaphylaxis and may require antihistamine or epinephrine to stop the reaction if bronchospasm occurs. The two most troublesome spiders in the United States are the black widow *(Latrodectus mactans)* and the brown recluse violin spider *(Loxosceles reclusa)*. The black widow's neurotoxin rarely results in death and confers lasting immunity against future bites but produces severe complications, including abdominal cramps, hypertension, reduced heartbeat, feeble pulse, shock, convulsions, and delirium. Bites by the brown recluse cause painful, spreading, slow-healing necrotic wounds that require medical attention. Very large doses of venom can cause hemolytic anemia, fever, jaundice, hematuria, and death.

Scorpion stings are especially dangerous to children under 5 years of age. Symptoms resemble those of strychnine poisoning and include pain, numbness, muscle spasm, blindness, and twitching of toes and fingers. Death results from respiratory paralysis. Centipedes and millipedes are not generally considered dangerous, but a few centipedes can inflict painful bites and some millipedes secrete a protective fluid that causes burns and brown discoloration to the skin.

Control of Arthropoda is difficult. Use of chemical sprays is widespread but has very serious consequences for the environment and other life forms because synthetic chemicals are not biodegradable and remain in the food chain. In addition, many insecticide-resistant species of insects have evolved. Other arthopod control methods being tried include increasing natural predators, destroying breeding grounds, biologic control (e.g., releasing artificially sterilized males, as was attempted with screwworm flies), pheromone and other types of trap bait, introduction of a faster-breeding competitive species, and removal of host species on which the insect feeds.

Basic morphologic differences among the classes and orders of arthropods make ticks, mites, flies, mosquitoes, bugs, lice, and fleas readily distinguishable from one another. The following section on insect morphology presents the major structural differences among the classes of medically important arthropods as well as some clinical and epidemiologic details. By studying Table 6–1, you can review those important genera of arthropods that transmit infections to humans.

GLOSSARY

Arthropoda. A phylum of the animal kingdom composed of organisms having a hard, segmented exoskeleton and paired, jointed legs.

Arachnida. A class in the phylum Arthropoda containing ticks, mites, spiders, and scorpions.

capitulum. A collective term referring to the mouthparts of ticks and mites that extend forward from the body of the tick or mite.

chitin. A horny, insoluble polysaccharide that is the main compound in shells of crabs, exoskeletons of insects, and other insect structures.

Crustacea. A class in the phylum Arthropoda including crabs, water fleas, lobsters, shrimp, barnacles, and wood lice.

ctenidium (pl. **ctenidia**). A spinelike process found on the head region of fleas. These comblike structures are useful in group classification. Genal ctenidia or combs are located just above the mouthparts. Pronotal combs are located immediately behind the head and extend posteriorly on the dorsal surface.

cypris. A larval resting stage in the life cycle of some crustaceans in which a metamorphosis occurs, comparable to a pupa.

ecdysis. The molting or shedding of an outer layer or covering and the development of a new one.

entomology. The branch of zoology dealing with the study of insects.

exoskeleton. A hard, chitinous structure on the outside of the body, providing support for internal organs.

imago. The sexually mature adult insect or arachnid.

Insecta. A class in the phylum Arthropoda containing many insect types whose bodies are divided into three distinct regions—head, thorax, and abdomen.

instar. Any one of the nymphal or larval stages between molts.

invertebrates. Animals having no spinal column.

metamorphosis. A change of shape or structure; a transition from one developmental stage to another. In simple or incomplete metamorphosis, nymphs resemble adults; in complete metamorphosis, larvae and pupae do not resemble adults.

myiasis. A condition caused by infestation of the body with fly larvae.

nauplius. The earliest and youngest larval form in the life cycle of crustaceans.

nymph. A developmental stage in the life cycle of certain arthropods that resembles the adult morphologically.

pediculosis. Infestation with lice, as with *Pediculus humanus.*

pupa (pl. **pupae**). The encased resting stage between the larva and imago stage (e.g., cocoon).

scutum. A chitinous shield or place covering part (female) or all (male) of the dorsal surface of hard ticks.

temporary host. A host on which an arthropod (adult or larval form) resides temporarily in order to feed on blood or tissue.

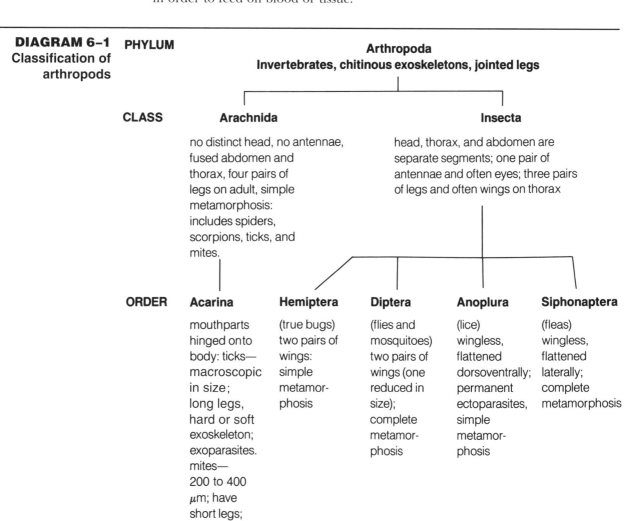

DIAGRAM 6–1
Classification of arthropods

PHYLUM

Arthropoda
Invertebrates, chitinous exoskeletons, jointed legs

CLASS

Arachnida

no distinct head, no antennae, fused abdomen and thorax, four pairs of legs on adult, simple metamorphosis: includes spiders, scorpions, ticks, and mites.

Insecta

head, thorax, and abdomen are separate segments; one pair of antennae and often eyes; three pairs of legs and often wings on thorax

ORDER

Acarina

mouthparts hinged onto body: ticks— macroscopic in size; long legs, hard or soft exoskeleton; exoparasites. mites— 200 to 400 μm; have short legs; endoparasities

Hemiptera

(true bugs) two pairs of wings: simple metamor- phosis

Diptera

(flies and mosquitoes) two pairs of wings (one reduced in size); complete metamor- phosis

Anoplura

(lice) wingless, flattened dorsoventrally; permanent ectoparasites, simple metamor- phosis

Siphonaptera

(fleas) wingless, flattened laterally; complete metamorphosis

INSECT MORPHOLOGY

Class Insecta

Order Diptera (Flies and Mosquitoes)

Diptera is the order of greatest medical importance; blood-sucking mosquitoes and flies transmit many viral, protozoan, and helminthic diseases. They are all ectoparasites as adults. One can differentiate among the dipteran insects by studying the characteristics of the parts listed and by using an identification key in an **entomology** text or insect identification handbook. Examine:

1. Antennae—number of segments, presence or absence of hairs
2. Mouth parts—structures for piercing skin or sucking fluid
3. Coloration and hair distribution on body
4. Size and shape of body and each of the three body segments—head, thorax, and abdomen
5. Morphology of egg, larval, and pupal stages
6. Pattern of veins in the wings

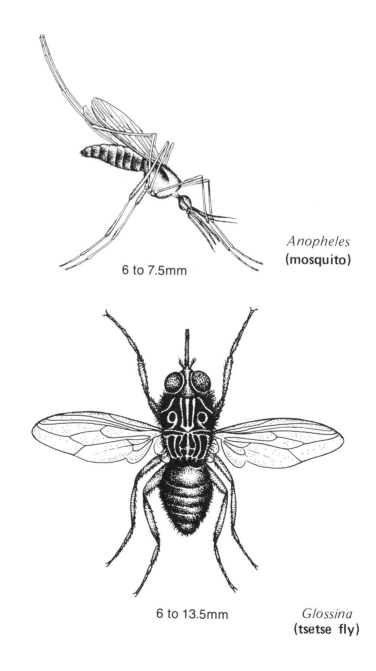

6 to 7.5mm

Anopheles
(mosquito)

6 to 13.5mm   *Glossina*
(tsetse fly)

Order Anoplura (Lice) Lice are flattened dorsoventrally and have a three-segment body with antennae on the head and three pairs of legs extending from the middle segment (the thorax). The legs have claws on the ends for grasping body hair. Metamorphosis is simple, and the immature stages look like the adults. Lice are very host-specific. The lice are permanent ectoparasites and live only on the host, surviving just briefly in the environment. Eggs (nits) are deposited on hair shafts of the host. The order Anoplura is blood-sucking lice; the mouthparts are adapted for piercing the skin and sucking blood. The head is narrower than the thorax; *Phthirus pubis* (crab louse) and *Pediculus humanus* (head and body lice) are epidemic in the United States, with·at least 6 million cases annually.

Lice are transferred directly from host to host. Additionally, eggs from louse-infested clothing or other personal articles may be sources of infection. Pubic lice are usually transferred via sexual intercourse, but infections may be acquired in locker rooms from towels and from mats on gymnasium floors. Symptoms of **pediculosis** include itchy papules at the site of infestation. Saliva and fecal excretions of the louse often cause a local hypersensitivity reaction that leads to inflammation. If secondary bacterial infection occurs, the lesion may resemble mange. Successful treatment requires that both eggs and motile stages be killed.

Body lice transmit *Rickettsia* spp., the causative agents of endemic typhus and trench fever. Louse-borne relapsing fever caused by *Borrelia recurrentis* is also transmitted by *P. humanus.*

Treatment. *P. pubis:* 0.5 percent malathion lotion or 1 percent lindane. *P. humanus:* (1) permethrin, (2) pyrethrin with butoxide or 0.5 percent malathion or 1 percent lindane.

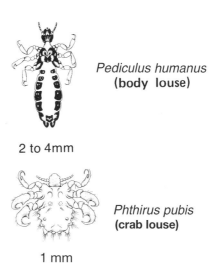

Pediculus humanus
(body louse)

2 to 4mm

Phthirus pubis
(crab louse)

1 mm

Order Siphonaptera (Fleas) Fleas are flattened laterally. They, too, have three pairs of clawed legs extending from the thorax, but the rear pair is very long and adapted for jumping. The species of fleas can be differentiated by looking for the presence or absence of eyes and the genal and pronotal **ctenidia** (combs). Adult fleas suck blood and have mouth parts adapted for this purpose. Metamorphosis is complete; all stages develop to maturity in the external environment. The adult flea takes a blood meal from a **temporary host** and then lays eggs in dark crevices. A flea infestation must be treated by cleaning the environment as well as the host. Complete chemical control is difficult. Chemical treatment and control measures in the environment should be repeated 2 weeks later to kill larvae and adults that develop from resistant eggs.

Adult fleas may live as long as a year, and eggs may remain viable for even longer periods. The rat flea, *Xenopsylla cheopis,* is known to transmit *Rickettsia typhi,* the bacteria responsible for murine typhus. The rat flea is the primary vector for the causative agent of bubonic plague, *Yersinia pestis.* Inasmuch as rats often live in colonies, fleas feed freely on various hosts. The disease is spread from rat to rat via flea bite. Infected fleas crushed on the host's body also allow the bacteria to gain entrance into the rat. Bubonic plague can be found in squirrels and other small mammals as well. Control of the disease rests mainly on controlling rats and squirrels. Under suitable conditions this bacteria may remain infective for 5 years in dried flea feces. These facts illustrate the difficulty of controlling fleas and the diseases they transmit.

As ectoparasites, fleas cause itchy bites when they feed. Adults usually feed several times in the same day and may move from host to host when several hosts are available. Furthermore, fleas are not very host-specific. Dog and cat fleas readily take a blood meal from humans. Although dog and cat fleas are not good transmitters of the plague bacillus, they can passively transmit tapeworms *(Hymenolepis nana* and *H. diminuta)* to humans. The primary problem caused by these fleas is irritation with possible allergic reactions to the bites. Secondary bacterial invasion may also occur as itchy bites are scratched.

Ctenocephalides spp.
(flea)

1.5 to 4mm

Class Arachnida

Order Acarina (Ticks and Mites)

The mouth parts of ticks and mites are adapted for piercing and are attached directly on the fused body. The mouth parts are part of an anterior structure known as a **capitulum,** which should be grasped firmly with forceps when removing an embedded tick to avoid leaving mouth parts in the skin. The thorax is fused to a globular body; head and antennae are absent. The adults have four pairs of legs. Acarid families include the following:

1. **Ixodidae**—a family containing the hard ticks that are temporary ectoparasites that feed on the host during larval, nymphal, and adult stages. Eggs are laid in the environment. Ticks can transmit several bacterial, rickettsial, viral, and at least one protozoal organism to humans, as noted in Table 6–1. Humans become infected with various organisms when the tick is feeding. Usually the pathogen enters the bloodstream directly, but it may also be rubbed into a wound if the area around the wound is contaminated with tick feces. An infected tick that has been crushed while being removed from people or pets may provide an additional source of infection. Furthermore, salivary secretions of some tick species can produce a toxemia (tick paralysis) that may result in death if the tick is not removed in time. And finally, bite wounds may become infected if mouth parts are left behind following tick removal. Ticks remain attached for extended feeding periods (up to several hours), and the local skin reaction to the mouth parts and the tick's salivary secretions becomes inflamed and is often accompanied by edema and hemorrhage.

   Adult ticks may live for 2 to 3 or more years and feed on several hosts. This longevity, coupled with the fact that most tick-borne organisms may be transmitted vertically (trans-stadial and/or transovarial passage), makes them very good vectors of disease.

2. **Argasidae**—a family containing the soft ticks that are also temporary ectoparasites. The body of soft ticks is soft and leathery, because it lacks the **scutum** found on the dorsal surface of hard ticks. They do not feed on humans.

3. **Sarcoptidae**—a family containing mites that are permanent ectoparasites that live and reproduce in burrows in the skin. Mites are quite host-specific and are usually transferred to new hosts in crowded quarters in which personal hygiene is neglected. Mites that normally infest other hosts may occasionally be temporary parasites of humans or other animals. For example, in the southern United States, *Ornithonyssus sylviarum*, a species of bird mite, migrates into homes from bird nests located in the eaves of houses. These insects attack cats, dogs, and humans, causing dermatitis, papules, vesicles, and even tissue necrosis at the bite site.

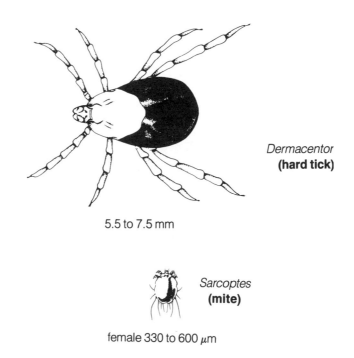

Dermacentor
(hard tick)

5.5 to 7.5 mm

Sarcoptes
(mite)

female 330 to 600 μm

The species *Sarcoptes scabiei* (the itch mite) causes the disease condition known as scabies (sarcoptic mange), which is diagnosed by finding the eggs, nymphs, or adults in skin scrapings of suspicious lesions. The diagnostic sign is a red tunnel measuring from a few millimeters to several centimeters in length, which turns into an extremely itchy papule. These mites have a relatively short life cycle, and newly hatched larvae reach adulthood in about 1 week. This short cycle allows infestations to become severe before treatment begins. *Sarcoptes scabiei* is endemic in the United States and elsewhere.

The morphologic characteristics of mites are similar to those in ticks except that mites are smaller and do not have a scutum. They are microscopic and their four pairs of legs are shorter, with only the two anterior pairs extending past the margins of the body.

Treatment. 1 percent lindane or 10 percent crotamiton

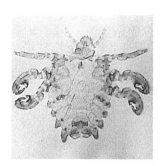
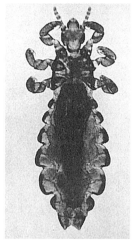
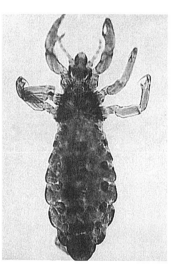
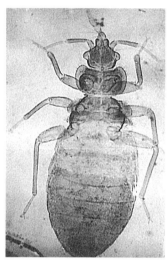
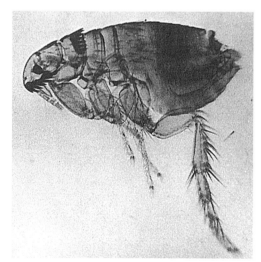
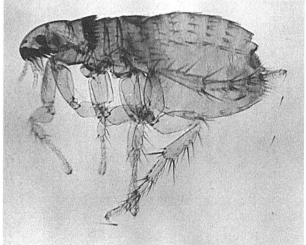

PHOTO 6–1 (*top left*). *Phthirus pubis* (crab louse), dorsal view (20×).

PHOTO 6–2 (*top right*). *Pediculus corporis* (Body louse), dorsal view (15×).

PHOTO 6–3 (*middle left*). *Pediculus capitis* (head louse), dorsal view (20×).

PHOTO 6–4 (*middle right*). *Cimex lectularius* (bedbug), dorsal view (20×).

PHOTO 6–5 (*bottom left*). *Ctenocephalides* spp. (male dog or cat flea), lateral view (15×).

PHOTO 6–6 (*bottom right*). *Ctenocephalides* spp. (female dog or cat flea), lateral view (15×).

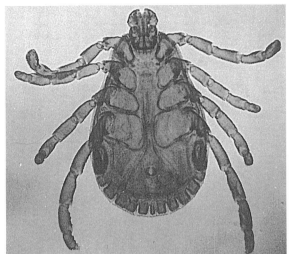

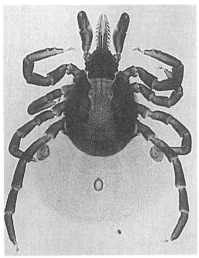

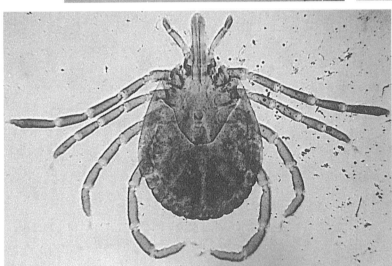

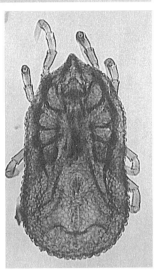

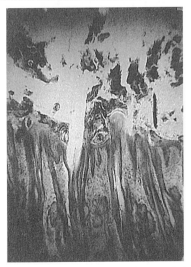

PHOTO 6–7 (*top left*). *Dermacentor andersoni* (hard tick), ventral view (10×).

PHOTO 6–8 (*top right*). *Ixodes* spp. (hard tick), dorsal view (20×).

PHOTO 6–9 (*middle left*). *Amblyomma americanum* (hard tick), dorsal view (10×).

PHOTO 6–10 (*middle right*). *Ornithodoros* spp. (soft tick), ventral view (10×).

PHOTO 6–11 (*bottom*). *Sarcoptes scabiei* (scabies in skin scraping) (40×).

Table 6–1. ARTHROPODS OF MEDICAL IMPORTANCE

Arthropod	Transmission Associations

Order Diptera (flies and mosquitoes)
  Family Culicidae (all mosquitoes)
    Aedes spp.
	1. Viral—encephalitis, yellow fever, dengue fever, hemorrhagic fever
	2. Nematoda—filariasis
	(*W. bancrofti*)

Anopheles spp.	1. Protozoa—malaria 2. Nematoda—filariasis (*W. bancrofti*—elephantiasis) (*B. malayi*) 3. Viral—various fevers and encephalitides
Culex spp.	1. Nematoda—filariasis (*W. bancrofti*) 2. Viral—encephalitis
Mansonia spp.	1. Nematoda—filariasis (*W. bancrofti*) (*B. malayi*) 2. Viral—various fevers
Family Ceratopogonidae (biting midges, punkies, no-see-ums) *Culicoides* spp.	1. Nematoda—filariasis (*M. ozzardi*) (*M. perstans*) (*M. streptocerca*)
Family Simuliidae (black flies, buffalo gnats) *Simulium* spp.	1. Nematoda—filariasis (*O. volvulus*) (*M. ozzardi*)
Family Psychodidae (sandfly) *Phlebotomus* spp.	1. Protozoa—leishmaniasis (*Leishmania* spp.)
Family Tabanidae (horse fly) *Tabanus* spp.	2. Viral—sandfly fever 3. Bacterial—*Bartonella bacilliformis* 1. Bacterial—anthrax and tularemia (*Bacillus anthracis*) (*Francisella tularensis*) 2. Protozoa—trypanosomes (mechanical transmission)
Chrysops spp. (mango fly) (deer fly)	1. Nematoda—filariasis (*Loa loa*)
Family Muscidae *Musca* spp. (house fly)	1. Bacterial—tularemia (*F. tularensis*) 2. Mechanical vector of many protozoan species
Stomoxys spp. (stable fly)	1. Mechanical vector of many protozoan species
Siphona spp. (horn fly)	1. Mechanical vector of many protozoan species
Glossina spp. (tsetse fly)	1. Mechanical vector of many protozoan species 2. Protozoa—trypanosomiasis (*Trypanosoma* spp.)
Other Fly Families *Cochliomyia* spp.	1. Myiasis—primary and secondary—screwworm
Other genera	1. Myiasis—maggots (fly larvae on skin wound)—warbles (fly larvae inside tissues)

Table 6–1. ARTHROPODS OF MEDICAL IMPORTANCE (Continued)

Arthropod	Transmission Associations

Order Hemiptera (bugs)
  Family Reduviidae
    Triatoma spp.
    Panstrongylus spp.
    (kissing bugs)
  Family Cimicidae
    Cimex spp.
    (bedbug)
	1. Protozoa—visceral trypanosomiasis *(T. cruzi)*
	
	1. Itchy bites

Order Siphonaptera (fleas)
  Family Pulicidae
    Xenopsylla spp.
    (Oriental rat flea)
 	
    Ctenocephalides spp.
    (cat or dog fleas)
	1. Bacterial—bubonic plague (black plague)
	   (Yersinia pestis)
	2. Cestoda
	   (H. nana)
	   (H. diminuta)
	3. Rickettsial—murine typhus
	   (Rickettsia mooseri)
	1. Cestoda
	   (D. caninum)

Order Parasitiformes
  Family Ixodidae
  (hard ticks)
    Dermacentor spp.
 	
    Ixodes spp.
	1. Rickettsial—Rocky Mountain spotted fever, Q fever
	   (R. rickettsii)
	   (Coxiella burnetti)
	2. Bacterial—tularemia
	   (F. tularensis)
	3. Viral—Colorado tick fever
	1. Protozoa—*Babesia* spp.
	2. Tick fever—*R. rickettsii*
	3. Viral—Colorado tick fever
	4. Spirochete—Lyme disease
	   (Borrelia burgdorferi)

Family Argasidae
(soft ticks)
    Ornithodoros spp.
 	
Family Sarcoptidae
(mites)
    Sarcoptes spp.
    (mange mite)
Family Trombiculidae
(mites)
    Trombicula spp.
    (chigger)
	1. Bacterial—Relapsing fever
	   (Borrelia recurrentis)
	
	1. Skin mange
	   (S. scabiei)
	
	1. Rickettsial—scrub typhus
	   (R. tsutsugamushi)

Order Anoplura (blood-sucking lice)
  Family Pediculidae
    Pediculus spp.
    (body lice)
 	
    Phthirus pubis
    (crab louse)
	1. Spirochetes—louse-borne relapsing fever
	   (B. recurrentis)
	2. Rickettsial—endemic typhus, trench fever
	   (R. prowazeki)
	   (R. quintana)
	1. Itchy bites

Table continued on following page

Table 6–1. ARTHROPODS OF MEDICAL IMPORTANCE (Continued)

Arthropod	Transmission Associations

Order Mallophaga (biting lice)
  Family Trichodectidae
    Trichodectes spp.
    (biting lice of domestic
    mammals)
	1. Cestoda—accidental infection
	   (*D. caninum*)
	   (*H. diminuta*)

Crustacea
Order Copepoda
  Cyclops spp.
  (copepod)
  (water flea)
 	
  Diaptomus spp.
  (copepod)
  (water flea)
Order Decapoda
  crayfish, crab
	1. Nematoda—Guinea worm
	   (*D. medinensis*)
	2. Cestoda—fish tapeworm
	   (*D. latum*)
	3. Sparganosis—*Spirometra* spp.
	1. Cestoda—fish tapeworm
	   (*D. latum*)
	
	1. Trematoda—lung fluke
	   (*P. westermani*)

You have now completed the section on Arthropoda. After reviewing this material with the aid of the learning objectives, proceed to the post-test.

BIBLIOGRAPHY

Alexander, JOD: Mites and skin diseases. Clinical Medicine 79:14, 1972.

Baker, EW, et al: *A Manual of Parasitic Mites of Medical or Economic Importance.* National Pest Control Association Technical Publication, New York, 1956.

Barnes, RD: *Invertebrate Zoology,* ed 3. WB Saunders, Philadelphia, 1974.

Beaver, PC, and Jung, RC: *Animal Agents and Vectors of Human Disease,* ed 5. Lea & Febiger, Philadelphia, 1985.

Belding, DL: *Textbook of Parasitology,* ed 3. Appleton-Century-Crofts, New York, 1965.

Borror, DJ, et al: *An Introduction to the Study of Insects,* ed 4. Holt, Rinehart & Winston, New York, 1976.

Brown, HW, and Neva, FA: *Basic Clinical Parasitology,* ed 5. Appleton-Century-Crofts, New York, 1983.

Burgess, I: *Sarcoptes scabiei* and Scabies. Adv Parasitol 33:235–292, 1994.

Davies, JE, Smith, RF, and Freed, V: Agromedical approach to pesticide management. Annu Rev Entomol 23:353, 1978.

Fain, A: The *Pentastomida* parasitic in man. Ann Soc Belg Med Trop 55:59, 1975.

Faust, EC, Beaver, PC, and Jung, RC: *Animal Agents and Vectors of Human Disease,* ed 4. Lea & Febiger, Philadelphia, 1975.

Fleas of Public Health Importance and Their Control. CDC-DHEW Publication, US Government Printing Office, Washington, DC, 1973.

Harves, AD, and Millikan, LE: Current concepts of therapy and pathophysiology in arthropod bites and stings, part 2. Insects: Review. Int J Dermatol 14:621, 1975.

Horen, PW: Insect and scorpion stings. JAMA 221:894, 1972.

Introduction to the Epidemiology of Vector-Borne Diseases, CDC-DHEW Publication, US Government Printing Office, Washington, DC, 1947.

James, MT: *The Flies That Cause Myiasis in Man.* Miscellaneous Publication No. 631, US. Government Printing Office, Washington, DC, 1960.

James, MT, and Harwood, RF: *Hermes' Medical Entomology,* ed 6. Macmillan, New York, 1969.

Lice of Public Health Importance and Their Control. CDC-DHEW Publication, US Government Printing Office, Washington, DC, 1973.

Orkin, J, Maibach, HI, and Parish, LC: *Scabies and Pediculosis.* JB Lippincott, Philadelphia, 1977.

Orlin, M, and Maibach, HI (eds): *Cutaneous Infestations and Insect Bites.* Marcel Dekker, New York, 1985.

Pest Control: An Assessment of Present and Alternative Technologies, Vol V. Pest Control and Health. Environmental Studies Board, National Research Council, National Academy of Science, Washington, DC, 1976.

Smart, J: *A Handbook for the Identification of Insects of Medical Importance.* British Museum, London, 1956.

Smith, KGV (ed): *Insects and Other Arthropods of Medical Importance.* British Museum (Natural History), London, 1973.

Sonenshine, DE: *Biology of Ticks,* Vol 2. Oxford University Press, New York, 1994.

Steere, AC, Broderick, TF, and Malawista, SE: Erythema chronicum migrans and Lyme arthritis: Epidemiologic evidence for a tick vector. Am J Epidemiol 108:312, 1978.

Ticks of Public Health Importance and Their Control. CDC-DHEW Publication, US Government Printing Office, Washington, DC, 1974.

Zumpt, F: *Myiasis in Man and Animals in the Old World: A Textbook for Physicians, Veterinarians, and Zoologists.* Butterworth, London, 1965.

POST-TEST

1. Matching: enter the single best number choice for parasite transmission: (**20 points**)

   a. _____ *Aedes*

   b. _____ *Anopheles*

   c. _____ *Simulium*

   d. _____ *Phlebotomus*

   e. _____ *Glossina*

   1. *Onchocerca volvulus*
   2. *Trypanosoma gambiense*
   3. *Leishmania b. donovani*
   4. *Giardia lamblia*
   5. *Brugia malayi*
   6. *Plasmodium vivax*

2. Indicate the type of Arthropoda that causes each of the following diseases or conditions. Use each number as many times as appropriate. (**40 points**)

   a. _____ myiasis

   b. _____ blood loss

   c. _____ crabs

   d. _____ scabies

   e. _____ sleeping sickness

   f. _____ babesiosis

   g. _____ Rocky Mountain spotted fever

   h. _____ Chagas' disease

   i. _____ the black plague

   j. _____ malaria

   1. bug
   2. mosquito
   3. tick
   4. louse
   5. fly
   6. mite
   7. flea

3. Based upon your knowledge of the life cycle of fleas and lice, discuss control measures necessary to prevent the spread of each. (**10 points**)

4. State at least five ways in which Arthropoda are harmful to humans. (**20 points**)

Each multiple choice question is worth **2 points.**

5. The arthropod vector associated with the transmission of the fish tapeworm is:
   a. *Aedes* spp.
   b. *Simulium* spp.
   c. *Phlebotomus* spp.
   d. *Cyclops* spp.
   e. *Pediculus* spp.

6. Obligate myiasis is associated with:
   a. *Triatoma* spp.
   b. *Cochliomyia* spp.
   c. *Cyclops* spp.
   d. *Glossina* spp.
   e. *Pediculus* spp.

7. Lyme disease is transmitted to humans by:
   a. *Ixodes* spp.
   b. *Dermacentor* spp.
   c. *Borrelia burgdorferi*
   d. *Mansonia* spp.
   e. *Phthirus pubis*

8. The nematode *Loa loa* is transmitted to humans by:
   a. *Triatoma* spp.
   b. *Sarcoptes* spp.
   c. *Musca* spp.
   d. *Mansonia* spp.
   e. *Chrysops* spp.

9. The mange mite is a:
   a. *Ornithodoros* spp.
   b. *Pediculus* spp.
   c. *Sarcoptes* spp.
   d. *Trichodectes* spp.
   e. *Trombicula* spp.

CHAPTER 7

Clinical Laboratory Procedures

LEARNING OBJECTIVES

Upon completion of this text and sufficient experience in a clinical parasitology laboratory, the student will be able to:

1   Recognize potential sources of error in laboratory procedures.
2   Recognize and sketch the important features of parasites present in clinical specimens that are routinely observed microscopically.
3   Calibrate and correctly use an ocular micrometer to measure parasites.
4   Demonstrate the proper technique for handling and disposing of contaminated materials.
5   State the proper procedures for collection and transport of fecal specimens.
6   Select proper procedures for performing a routine fecal analysis for the presence of parasitic infections.
7   Properly prepare fecal smears.
8   Properly prepare iodine-stained and unstained wet mounts of fecal material.
9   Correctly perform the trichrome stain on fecal material.
10 Properly scan a microscope slide for the presence of parasites and identify by scientific name all parasites found therein.
11 Select appropriate concentration technique for the recovery of any given parasite.
12 Correctly perform the zinc sulfate flotation and the formalin-ethyl acetate sedimentation concentration techniques for recovery of intestinal parasites.
13 Correctly prepare thin and thick blood smears.
14 Correctly perform the Giemsa staining technique for blood smears.
15 Identify parasites in a stained blood smear.
16 Select proper procedures and protocol for the identification of Filaria infections.
17 Identify parasites present on a cellophane tape preparation for pinworms.
18 Prepare and maintain in vitro cultures of protozoa.
19 Correctly and accurately perform a fecal egg count.
20 Prepare all solutions used routinely in the laboratory.
21 Prepare serum for parasite serology.
22 Correctly perform and evaluate serologic tests for parasitic infections.
23 Demonstrate correct procedures and protocol for quality control measures.

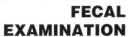

FECAL EXAMINATION   General considerations for a routine fecal examination in the clinical laboratory include the following:

1. Naturally passed stools are preferred for examination. Specimens can be passed into a clean, widemouthed cardboard container or bedpan. Samples collected in a bedpan **must not** be contaminated with urine and must be transferred to an appropriate container before being submitted to the laboratory. All specimens must be correctly and completely labeled. Appropriate labeling requires at least the following information: the patient's name, hospital or other identification number, attending physician's name, date and time of collection, and the time of specimen arrival in the laboratory. Because specimens may also be infected with other pathogens such as viruses, fungi, or bacteria, it is best to place all specimen containers in plastic zipper-locking bags before delivering them to the laboratory so that all workers handling the samples are adequately protected from infective agents.

2. For a routine parasitic workup, it is recommended that patients submit two normal movements, one every other day, and that a third specimen be obtained by using a cathartic such as Epsom salt (magnesium sulfate) or Fleet Phospho-Soda. The purged specimen is unnecessary if the patient already has diarrhea.

   NOTE: One or two specimens are often sufficient for the recovery and identification of helminth eggs.

3. An initial examination of fresh specimens should be made according to the following guideline: liquid within 30 minutes, semisolid within 1 hour, and formed within 24 hours of collection. Formed stools may be refrigerated for 1 to 2 days if their examination must be delayed, although this practice does not guarantee the recovery of all parasites. If examination must be delayed more than 24 hours, the specimen should be preserved in polyvinyl alcohol (PVA) or formalin. Hookworm eggs mature and hatch if allowed to remain at room temperature and may be confused with *Strongyloides* larvae unless carefully observed. (See also page 132 for transport procedures.)

4. Protozoan cysts may be found more commonly in formed stools and are often easier to identify than trophozoites. Trophozoites are found more commonly in liquid stools or those obtained by saline purgation. Because trophozoites do not survive for great lengths of time and their motility is of diagnostic importance, specimens must be examined in a timely manner. For this reason, **it is important to require and verify collection and arrival times for all fecal specimens**; otherwise, reported results may be invalid. If transportation to the laboratory is to be delayed, part of the specimen should be preserved, when collected, in PVA-fixative* or in 10 percent aqueous formalin.* Formalin preserves eggs, cysts, and larvae for wet-mount examination and for concentration. PVA-fixative preserves cysts and trophozoites for permanent staining.

5. When amebiasis or giardiasis is suspected, several specimens (at least three) should be examined, one every other day. Additional specimens are examined when necessary. For each specimen received, a permanently stained slide should be prepared and examined. Purged specimens must be examined immediately or they are worthless. Saline purges using Epsom salt, sodium sulfate, or Fleet Phospho-Soda are satisfactory, but castor oil, mineral oil, or suppositories make examination for protozoa impossible.

6. Feces containing x-ray contrast media, such as barium salts, are to be rejected because these make a proper examination impossible. If barium salts have been given, it is necessary to wait from 5 to 10 days before submitting a specimen for parasitic examination.

7. All specimens for parasitic studies should be collected before beginning treatment with any antibiotics, but if antibiotics have been given, new fecal collections should not begin until 2 weeks after therapy has ended.

---

*Methods of preparation of reagents noted in this chapter and marked by asterisks are described on pages 140–143.

8. For growth of *Entamoeba histolytica*, culture media such as Balamuth, Boeck and Drbohlav, McQuay, or Cleveland-Collier may be useful. Various authorities express conflicting views on the relative usefulness of culture media, inasmuch as the number of cysts needed for viable cultures may be so great that they should be detectable at that number in feces by ordinary microscopic methods.

9. The Occupational Safety and Health Administration's (OSHA) Final Rule on Bloodborne Pathogens required that all laboratories were to be in compliance with its rule by July 6, 1992. In part, the rule states that:

> The standard for reducing worker exposure to bloodborne pathogens is based on the adoption of universal precautions as a method of infection control. This approach assumes that all human blood and body fluids are potentially infectious for HIV (human immunodeficiency virus), HBV (hepatitis B virus), and other bloodborne pathogens.
>
> Universal Precautions is defined as a method of infection control in which all human blood and certain body fluids are treated as if known to be infectious for HIV, HBV, and other bloodborne pathogens.

While the rule does not specifically refer to parasitic diseases found in other body locations, the procedures needed to protect a worker from bloodborne pathogens provide protection from virtually all infectious agents. From other information presented in the OSHA ruling, the following specific safety guidelines are suggested:

A. Gloves and a protective coat or apron must be worn when handling feces or other specimens.
B. Hands should be washed with disinfectant soap on entering the laboratory and after removing gloves.
C. Laboratory garments should never be worn outside the laboratory.
D. Nothing should be placed in the mouth when in the laboratory.
E. Avoid touching your face with your hands, and do not place personal articles such as eyeglasses or books on the workbench.
F. Care should be taken to maintain all working space in a neat and clean condition. The workbench should be cleaned with disinfectant such as 2.5 percent Amphyl (soap, *o*-phenylphenol, and alcohol) or a 50 percent bleach solution made with water and commercial bleach before and after each work period.
G. All contaminated materials should immediately be placed in a disinfectant or other appropriate container for disposal.
H. Spills should be overlaid with Amphyl or a 50 percent commercial bleach solution and absorbent towels or sand. After 10 minutes, dispose of the contaminated material in a plastic biohazard bag or other suitable container.
I. If spills create aerosols, especially from a centrifuge accident, all personnel should leave the laboratory at once for 1 hour. The person responsible for cleaning up the spill should wear protective clothing, gloves, and mask.

MACROSCOPIC EXAMINATION

The process of macroscopic examination, a routine component of a fecal examination for parasites, involves the following procedures:

1. Note the consistency of the specimen. Mushy or liquid stools suggest the possible presence of trophozoites or intestinal protozoa. Protozoan cysts are found more frequently in formed stools. Helminth eggs and larvae may be found in either liquid or formed stools.
2. Examine the surface of the specimen for parasites (e.g., tapeworm proglottids or, less commonly, adult pinworms).
3. Break up the stool with applicator sticks to check for the presence of adult helminths (e.g., *Ascaris*).

4. Examine the stool for blood and/or mucus.
   a. Fresh blood (bright red) indicates acute lower intestinal tract bleeding.
   b. Bloody mucus suggests ulceration, and some of this material should be preferentially examined microscopically for trophozoites.
5. Feces should be sieved after drug treatment for tapeworms to ensure recovery of the scolex.

Of Note

1. Adult worms, if recovered, are examined and identified directly.
2. Tapeworms are speciated by examining gravid proglottids. Because eggs of *T. solium* are infective for humans, great care must be exercised when handling these specimens. When examining a gravid proglottid, it should be fixed in 10 percent formalin and then cleared by immersing it in glycerin or lactophenol solution (1:1). Uterine branches may be made more visible by injecting a small amount of India ink into the uterine or genital pore. A 1-mL syringe with a 25-gauge needle should be used to inject the ink. The segment should then be flattened by gently pressing it between two glass slides.

MICROSCOPIC EXAMINATION

The routine examination of fecal specimens for "ova and parasites" consists of three distinct procedures, including a direct wet mount, a fecal concentration technique, and a permanently stained fecal smear. The direct wet mount is a rapid-screening technique and is used to study trophozoite motility. The concentration method increases the chance for recovering parasitic forms, and the various staining procedures are used to study and confirm the identity of small parasites such as protozoa. Each of these procedures is described below.

Direct Wet Mount

Direct wet mounts are prepared by using an applicator stick to thoroughly mix a small amount of feces with a drop of saline placed on a microscope slide. Apply a 22-mm cover glass so that air bubbles are not trapped under the glass. A smear should be thin enough that a printed page can be read through it. The entire preparation must be examined for the presence of eggs, larvae, and protozoa. Systematic examination, using the 10× lens, may be accomplished by starting at the lower edge of the slide and observing each field until the upper edge is reached (Diagram 7–1). Then move the preparation one field to the right and examine each field downward until the lower edge is reached. Move right one field and continue in this manner until the entire slide has been examined. Next, several random fields should be examined using the high dry objective lens, inasmuch as protozoa may have been overlooked at 10× magnification. Care must be exercised when adjusting the light on the microscope. A common error is the use of too much light, which prevents proper contrast. Because protozoa are translucent and col-

DIAGRAM 7–1

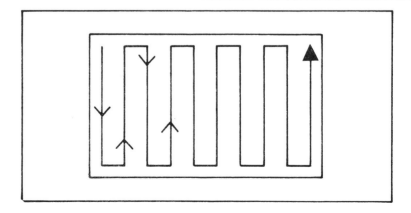

orless when unstained, they are not visible unless the light is reduced. Iodine* may be used to help demonstrate eggs and cyst structures more clearly, but this kills and distorts trophozoites so that motility cannot be observed. A saline mount and an iodine mount may be prepared at opposite ends of the same slide, using separate coverslips.

A calibrated ocular micrometer should be used routinely. Size differences of various internal structures and of whole organisms are important in differential diagnosis.

1. Install an ocular micrometer disk in the eyepiece of the microscope by placing it underneath the eyepiece lens.
2. Place a stage micrometer on the microscope's stage and, using the 10× objective, focus on the stage scale. The stage scale is 1 mm long and is calibrated in hundredths; each .01 mm = 10 μm.
3. Line up the left edge of the ocular scale with the left edge of the stage scale (Diagram 7–2).
4. Find a place at the farthest point to the right where a line on the ocular micrometer is exactly superimposed on a line of the stage micrometer.
5. The number of micrometers indicated by each division on the ocular scale can be calculated using the following formula:

$$\frac{\text{Number of stage micrometer spaces} \times 10 \ \mu m}{\text{Number of ocular micrometer spaces}} = \mu m/\text{ocular space}$$

Example: In Diagram 7–2, note that the 40th ocular scale line is exactly superimposed over the 30th stage scale line (0.3 mm). Using the formula: 30 × 10/40 = 7.5 μm/ocular space.

6. Steps 2 through 6 must be repeated for each objective lens. Record the calibration equivalent for each objective so that parasites may be measured when viewed at any magnification. It is convenient to post these values on the microscope.
7. To measure a parasite, line up one edge of the egg or cyst with the zero on the ocular scale, count the number of ocular spaces to the other edge, and multiply by the appropriate lens factor (e.g., × 7.5 μm in the previous example).

DIAGRAM 7–2

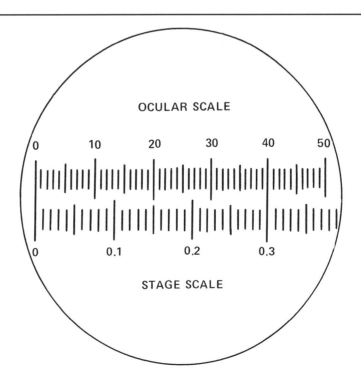

Results and Report for Direct Wet Mounts

1. Any observed parasites are reported by their scientific name, including both the genus and species names when possible, and the specific stage (e.g., eggs, trophozoites, larvae).
2. Certain cellular elements, such as blood cells or yeast, and *Blastocystis hominis* should be reported semiquantitatively as few, moderate, or many RBCs, WBCs, yeast, or other cells if they are clearly identifiable. *Trichuris trichiura* and trematode infections should also be quantitated in this manner.
3. Charcot-Leyden crystals may be reported semiquantitatively as few, moderate, or many Charcot-Leyden crystals.

Of Note

1. Many artifacts and other formed structures can be seen when examining a wet mount. These include red blood cells, white blood cells, macrophages, mucosal epithelium, yeast, undigested vegetable cells, pollen grains, and hair. To the untrained eye, any of these may be mistaken for parasites. It is important to be familiar with these artifacts.
2. Eosinophils may be present, indicating an allergic immune response that may be related to a parasitic infection or to another allergen such as pollen or food. Breakdown products of degenerating eosinophils form Charcot-Leyden crystals, which appear as slender crystals with pointed ends and stain red-purple with trichrome stain. Their presence indicates that an allergic immune response has occurred.
3. Free-living ameba, flagellates, or even ciliates may be found in specimens that have been contaminated with water from sewage, stagnant ponds, or soil. These organisms may be quite difficult to differentiate from pathogens.
4. Wet mounts for screening can also be made from fecal specimens preserved in formalin or PVA, but no motility of organisms will be present and this step can be omitted if this is the only specimen received.

Quality Control Considerations

1. Verify weekly that the iodine solution is clear and not contaminated with bacteria or fungus and that it has the dark brown color of strong tea.
2. Positive control material can be prepared by adding fixed human buffy coat cells to negative stool specimens. The cytoplasm of white blood cells has a yellow-gold color, similar to that of protozoan trophozoites. A preserved known-positive fecal specimen can also be used for quality control (QC). The control specimen should be examined at least quarterly or whenever new stain is prepared.
3. The ocular micrometer and microscope should be calibrated at least annually.
4. Quality control results should be recorded, and the action plan for "out of control" results should be followed if needed.
5. The laboratory name should also be on the report.

CONCENTRATION TECHNIQUES FOR PARASITE STAGES IN FECES

A fecal concentration technique increases the possibility of detecting parasites when few are present in feces and is a routine part of the clinical procedures. A single concentrate from one fecal specimen is frequently sufficient to detect clinically important infections.

Two general types of methods are used—sedimentation and flotation. The formalin-ethyl acetate sedimentation concentration method, a modification of the formalin-ether method of Ritchie, is the most commonly used technique for concentrating eggs and cysts and is more efficient than flotation methods.

Sedimentation Method

Procedure for the Formalin-Ethyl Acetate Method. This method concentrates parasite stages present in a large amount of feces into about 2 g of sediment.

1. 5 to 15 g (½ to 1 teaspoon) of fresh feces is added to a suitable container and is mixed well with 10 to 15 mL of 10 percent formalin using applicator sticks. Allow the mixture to stand for 30 minutes for fixation. This step kills and preserves pro-

tozoa, larvae, and most eggs. Some eggshells, such as *Ascaris*, are impervious to formalin.

2. Strain the mixture through two layers of dampened surgical gauze into a 15-mL conical centrifuge tube and add enough formalin to nearly fill the tube.

   a. Do not use more than two layers of surgical gauze or more than one layer of the newer "pressed" gauze because thicker layers trap mucus containing *Cryptosporidium* spp. oocysts or microsporidia.

   b. Do not strain any specimen that contains a large amount of mucus. Instead, centrifuge the mixture for 10 minutes at 500*g*, decant into disinfectant, and continue the procedure with Step 7.

3. The suspension is centrifuged at 500*g* (1500 rpms) for 10 minutes. The supernatant is decanted into disinfectant. The sediment is resuspended in saline or formalin and recentrifuged if the sample contains excessive debris. (The rpms are noted so that workers may more easily adjust speeds to the appropriate gravity when using common tabletop centrifuges, but proper calibration steps should be performed to verify speeds.)

4. Resuspend the washed stool sediment in 7 mL of 10 percent formalin and add 4 mL of ethyl acetate. Stopper the tube and shake it vigorously for 30 seconds. Carefully remove the stopper away from the face as organic vapor may cause spurting of fecal debris. This step extracts fats from the feces and reduces bulk; do not use if a very small amount of debris is present or if the original specimen contains a lot of mucus.

5. Centrifuge the tube for 10 minutes at 500*g*. Four layers should result.

6. After the upper debris layer has been rimmed with an applicator stick (Diagram 7–3), the entire supernatant is decanted into disinfectant. Invert the centrifuge tube completely in one smooth motion, but only once. If excess ethyl acetate is left inside the tube or if the tube is plastic, a cotton-tipped applicator stick should be used to swab the inside of the tube while the tube is still inverted. Excess ethyl acetate appears as bubbles when the slide preparation is made and may dissolve plastic tubes.

7. A small drop of fecal sediment and 1 drop of iodine stain are then mixed together on a slide. A cover glass is added, and the entire preparation is examined carefully for parasites. An unstained preparation also should be examined, because cysts are refractile and more easily detected unstained, and also because the morphology of unstained larval forms is more characteristic.

DIAGRAM 7–3

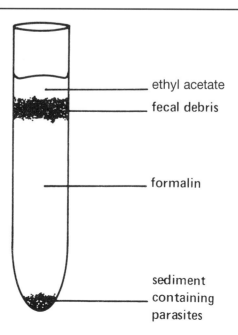

ethyl acetate

fecal debris

formalin

sediment
containing
parasites

Of Note

1. Ethyl acetate has replaced the use of ether. Ethyl acetate is nonflammable; therefore, it is a much safer chemical for laboratory use. Recovery of *Hymenolepis nana* eggs and cysts of *Giardia lamblia* is enhanced with this reagent. Some workers consider Hemo De to be even safer than ethyl acetate.
2. Centrifugation speeds and times are important because recovery of *Crytosporidium* oocysts may be missed if centrifugation is insufficient.
3. If water is used as a rinsing fluid in Step 3, *Blastocystis hominis* cysts rupture, leading to a false-negative report for this organism.
4. The sedimentation procedure can be used to concentrate PVA-fixed material as follows: Thoroughly mix the PVA-stool suspension with applicator sticks, add about 4 mL of the mixture to a test tube containing 10 mL of saline, and mix well. Filter the mixture through gauze as in Step 2 and continue the procedure as described. SAF-preserved specimens can be processed beginning directly at Step 2. *Isospora belli* is often missed in PVA-preserved concentrates.
5. Extra washing of fixed sediment may be necessary, because iodine causes precipitation of excess mercuric chloride. If precipitation is noted when the slide is examined, simply rewash the sediment once or twice and prepare a new slide. Some authorities do not recommend concentrating PVA-fixed materials because protozoa become so distorted that they are not recognizable.

Results and Report for Sedimentation Procedures

1. Any observed parasites are reported by their scientific name, including both the genus and species names when possible, and the stage present.
2. Certain cellular elements such as blood cells or yeast may be reported semiquantitatively as few, moderate, or many RBCs, WBCs, yeast, or other cells if they are clearly identifiable.
3. Charcot-Leyden crystals may be reported semiquantitatively as few, moderate, or many Charcot-Leyden crystals.

Quality Control Considerations

1. Verify weekly that all solutions are clear and are not visibly contaminated.
2. Known positive specimens should be concentrated and organisms should be identified to verify technique at least quarterly or whenever the centrifuge has been calibrated.
3. Quality control results should be recorded and the action plan for "out of control" results should be followed if needed.

Flotation Methods

Flotation methods use liquids with a higher specific gravity than that of eggs or cysts so that parasites float to the surface and can then be skimmed from the top of the tube. The concentrating solution should have a final specific gravity of 1.18 (1.20 can be used with preserved specimens). The most commonly used reagent is zinc sulfate, and a description of the procedure using this solution follows. It is important to note that operculated eggs as well as schistosome and infertile ascaris eggs are not easily recovered by this method. In addition, the high specific gravity kills trophozoites and causes distortion of certain other fragile eggs, such as *Hymenolepis nana*. For these reasons, it is recommended that if only a single concentration procedure is used, it should be the formalin-ethyl acetate sedimentation technique.

Procedure for the Zinc Sulfate* Flotation Method. The procedure should be accomplished as follows:

1. Prepare washed feces in a 13 × 100-mm round-bottom tube as described in Steps 1 and 2 of the procedure for the formalin-ethyl acetate concentration method.
2. Wash once or twice in saline (centrifuge each time at $500g$ [1500 rpm] for 10 minutes) to obtain 1 mL or less of sediment.
3. Resuspend and thoroughly mix the sediment in 12 mL of zinc sulfate solution (specific gravity 1.18 to 1.20 as verified with a hydrometer).

DIAGRAM 7–4

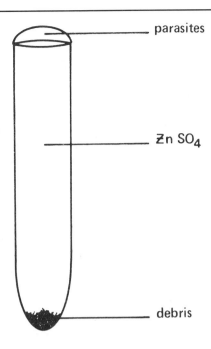

parasites

$Zn\ SO_4$

debris

4. Centrifuge for 2 minutes at $500g$ (1500 rpm), allowing the centrifuge to stop without vibration. Place tube in a rack in a vertical position without shaking it, and slowly add enough zinc sulfate down the side of the tube with a dropper pipette to fill the tube so that an inverted meniscus forms (Diagram 7–4).
5. Without shaking the tube, carefully place a 22×22-mm cover glass on top of the tube so that its underside rests on the meniscus. The meniscus should not be so high that fluid runs down the side of the tube, carrying parasitic forms away from the cover glass.
6. Allow the tube to stand vertically in a rack with the coverslip suspended on top for 10 minutes.
7. Carefully lift the cover glass with its hanging drop containing parasites on the underside and mount on a clean slide, liquid side down. A small drop of iodine stain may be placed on the slide prior to adding the cover glass. The slide is gently rotated after adding the cover glass to ensure a uniform mixture. The coverslip preparation is thoroughly examined microscopically, using the procedure outlined on page 124.

Of Note   Gravity flotation is not particularly effective in concentrating organisms. Many workers prefer the following variation:

1. After washing as in Step 1, resuspend sediment in 12 mL of zinc sulfate solution. Then fill the tube to within 0.5 mL of its top.
2. Centrifuge for 2 minutes at $500g$ (1500 rpm) and allow the centrifuge to stop without vibration.
3. Use either a sterile Pasteur pipette or a flamed and cooled wire loop (bent at a right angle to the stem) to transfer 2 or 3 drops of the surface film to a clean glass slide. Add a drop of iodine stain, mix, and add a cover glass. Examine microscopically.
4. Oocysts of *Isospora belli* and some other organisms are so lightweight that they float very near the top of the liquid. It is important not to allow liquid to run down the side of the tube when placing a coverslip on top of the tube in Step 1. For the same reason, it is important to skim the top of the meniscus when using a wire loop as mentioned.

5. Some thin-shelled helminth eggs and protozoan cysts are distorted by prolonged exposure to the high specific gravity of the zinc sulfate solution, so microscopic examination of these samples must be done promptly.
6. If flotation is the only concentration technique used, the sediment should also be examined.

Results and Report for Flotation Procedures

1. Any observed parasites are reported by their scientific name, including both the genus and species names when possible.
2. Certain cellular elements such as blood cells or yeast may be reported semiquantitatively as few, moderate, or many RBCs, WBCs, yeast, or other cells if they are clearly identifiable.
3. Charcot-Leyden crystals may be reported semiquantitatively as few, moderate, or many Charcot-Leyden crystals.

Quality Control Considerations

1. Verify weekly that all solutions are clear and are not visibly contaminated.
2. Known positive specimens should be concentrated and organisms should be identified to verify technique at least quarterly or whenever the centrifuge has been calibrated.
3. The ocular micrometer and microscope should be calibrated at least annually.
4. Quality control results should be recorded and the action plan for "out of control" results should be followed if needed.

TRICHROME STAIN FOR INTESTINAL PROTOZOA

The Wheatley trichrome* technique is a rapid procedure giving good results for routine identification of intestinal protozoa in fresh fecal specimens. It is considered to be the final part of a complete fecal examination. This procedure is the confirmation step for all identifications of protozoan parasites, even if parasites are identified earlier. Smaller protozoans such as microsporidia may be missed completely if this step is omitted.

The cytoplasm of *E. histolytica* trophozoites and cysts appears light blue-green or light pink. *E. coli* cysts are slightly more purple. Nuclear structure is clearly visible; karyosomes of nuclei stain ruby red. Degenerated organisms stain pale green. Background material stains green, providing a good contrast with the protozoa. The procedure requires that fecal smears be fixed with either PVA* or Schaudinn* solution.

1. Using an applicator stick, place a thin film of fresh feces on a microscope slide and, while the smear is wet, place it in Schaudinn fixative (without acetic acid) for 5 minutes at 50°C or 1 hour at room temperature. Rinse in 70 percent alcohol for 5 minutes to remove excess fixative. (Omit this fixation if smears have been preserved in PVA.) Diarrheic stools should be mixed with PVA fixative. The fixative acts as an adhesive. When using PVA-fixed material from a transport vial, the following procedure should be followed:
   a. Using an applicator stick, spread some of the specimen onto a clean glass slide. Adherence to the slide is improved if the material is spread to the edges of the slide.
   b. Slides should be dried either for several hours at room temperature, or for 1 to 2 hours on a slide warmer or in a 37°C incubator. Morphologic distortion may result if slides are dried too rapidly. The slide must be dried thoroughly to avoid washing off the film during staining.
2. Place slide in the 70 percent ethanol solution (with enough iodine added to turn the alcohol to the color of strong tea) for 2 minutes (10 minutes for PVA-fixed smears).
3. Place slide successively in two changes of 70 percent solutions of ethanol for 5 minutes in each solution. Place in trichrome* stain for 10 to 20 minutes.
4. Rinse in acidified 90 percent ethanol* for 10 to 20 seconds. Usually a brief dip in and out is sufficient.

   NOTE: Inasmuch as the acid alcohol continues to destain as long as it is in contact with the material, the time allowed should include the few seconds between the time the slide is removed from the destain and the subsequent rinse in absolute alcohol in Step 6.

5. Rinse quickly with several dips each in two changes of absolute ethanol. These alcohol solutions should be changed frequently to prevent them from becoming so acid that the destaining process continues. Prolonged destaining in acid alcohol (more than 20 seconds) may cause the organisms to be poorly differentiated. Larger trophozoites, particularly those of *E. coli*, may require slightly longer periods of decolorization.

   NOTE: If several slides are stained simultaneously, they should be destained separately. Remove only one slide at a time from the stain. Destain it, rinse it in the 100 percent alcohols, and continue with Step 7.

6. Place in two changes of absolute ethanol for 5 minutes each.
7. Place in clear xylene (or xylene substitute) for 5 minutes.
8. Mount with a cover glass, using balsam or another mounting medium.
9. Examine under oil immersion as described previously.

Results and Report for the Trichrome Stain Procedure

1. Trophozoites and cysts, human tissue or blood cells, and yeast (single, budding, or pseudohyphae) are easily identified, but helminth eggs and larvae often retain excessive stain, making them difficult to identify.
2. Any observed parasites are reported by their scientific names, including both the genus and species names when possible, and stage.
3. Certain cellular elements such as blood cells or yeast may be reported semiquantitatively as few, moderate, or many RBCs, WBCs, yeast, or other cells such as macrophages if they are clearly identifiable.
4. Charcot-Leyden crystals may be reported semiquantitatively as few, moderate, or many Charcot-Leyden crystals.
5. All reportable objects may be quantitated using the following scheme:

Number of Organisms, Cells, or Other Artifacts Counted in 10 Oil Immersion Fields	Quantity Reported
≤ 2	Few
3–9	Moderate
≥ 10	Many

Quality Control Considerations

1. Since trichrome stains are quite stable, it is usually necessary only to check each new batch of stain. If staining is done very infrequently, it is advisable that periodic checks be made, at least monthly.
2. Positive control material can be prepared by adding human buffy coat cells to negative stool specimens. From this mixture, smears are made and stained along with unknown slides. Known negative slides should be processed with each set of unknowns. If positive fecal material is available from patients or quality control survey samples, control slides may be made from PVA-fixed material. Check white blood cells and known parasites for color.
3. The ocular micrometer and microscope should be calibrated at least annually.
4. The 70 percent ethanol-iodine solution should be changed at least weekly or more frequently if slides are too green.
5. Quality control results should be recorded and the action plan for "out of control" results should be followed if needed.

OTHER DIAGNOSTIC PROCEDURES

Several other procedures are commonly used in the laboratory and are presented in this section in order of frequency.

SPECIMEN TRANSPORT PROCEDURES

Many laboratories in small hospitals, private clinics, or physicians' offices do not routinely perform examinations for eggs and parasites. These laboratories must send specimens to larger laboratories. Successful diagnosis of intestinal parasitic diseases requires "fresh" stool specimens. When examinations must be delayed, it is important to preserve specimen integrity by placing it in a proper transport medium.

A two-vial system is currently accepted as a standard means of transport. One vial should contain 8 to 10 mL of polyvinyl alcohol (PVA) fixative,* and a second vial should contain 8 to 10 mL of 10 percent formalin. To each vial, 2 to 3 mL of feces is added. Be sure to select appropriate (e.g., bloody, slimy, or watery) specimen areas. Sample material should be taken from the outer edge, ends, and middle of formed stools. Thoroughly mix the sample using applicator sticks. Cap the vial tightly. The specimen is now ready for transport. Additionally, a 2-mL sample of feces may be placed in a clean, empty vial so that other examinations such as ameba culture or the rearing of hookworm larvae may be performed.

The receiving laboratory then processes the sample. Smears for trichrome* staining should be made from the PVA tube. Direct wet mounts made from the 10 percent formalin vial can be examined, and either tube may be used as source material for the formalin-ethyl acetate concentration method. The zinc sulfate flotation method can be performed using the 10 percent formalin vial.

CELLOPHANE TAPE TEST FOR PINWORM

As the female pinworm *(Enterobius vermicularis)* migrates out of the anus to deposit her eggs on the perianal region, eggs may be easily recovered there for identification. A parent can collect the specimen from a young child at home using a kit supplied by the doctor.

Procedure. The following test should be performed in the morning before the patient has washed or defecated, because the eggs are generally deposited in the perianal region at night.

1. Fold the edges of a 3 × ¾-inch piece of clear cellophane tape around the end of a tongue depressor so that the sticky side is out.
2. Spread the buttocks and apply the tape face to the anal area, using a rocking motion to touch as much of the perianal mucosa as possible.
3. Remove the tape and apply it to a microscope slide, sticky side down. Press firmly so that no air bubbles are trapped (Diagram 7–5).
4. Examine the slide for pinworm eggs under low power using low light as described

DIAGRAM 7–5

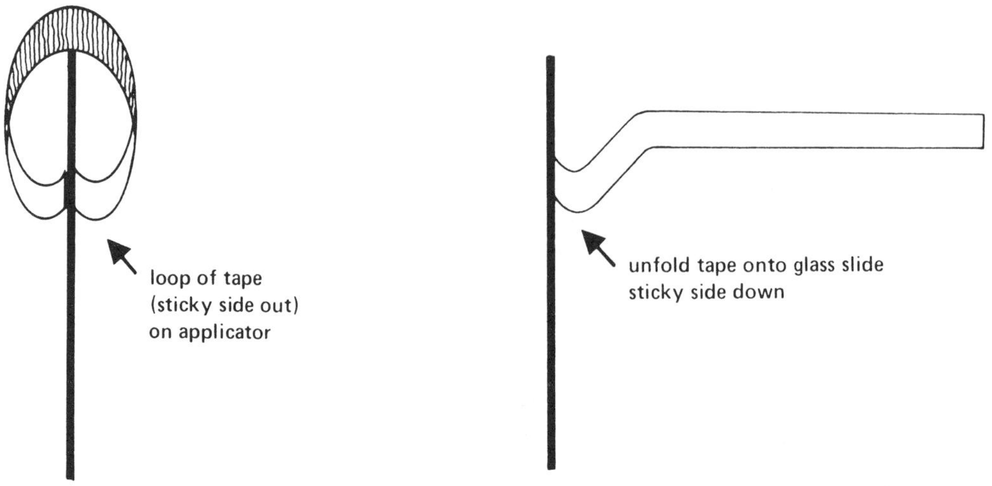

loop of tape
(sticky side out)
on applicator

unfold tape onto glass slide
sticky side down

in the microscopic examination on page 124. Be sure to examine the entire area under the tape. The eggs are colorless; therefore, good focus and low-light contrast are critical.

Of Note

1. Pinworm infection should not be ruled out until at least five daily consecutive negative preparations have been examined.
2. Cellophane tape can be cleared by lifting one edge of the tape from the slide and then placing 1 or 2 drops of xylol or toluol under the tape before examination. Disperse the liquid by carefully pressing the tape down onto the slide.

Results and Report for Cellophane Tape Preparation

Pinworm eggs are reported as found or not found.

MODIFIED KINYOUN ACID-FAST STAIN (COLD METHOD)

In recent years, *Cryptosporidium parvum, I. belli,* and the microsporidia have caused severe diarrheal diseases in immunocompromised patients. Because these parasites may be difficult to detect and identify by routine methods, it is necessary to use the acid-fast stain method to confirm their identity.

This procedure may be used on fresh, formalin-preserved or SAF-preserved fecal sediment or on other clinical specimens such as duodenal fluid, bile, or any type of pulmonary specimen. PVA-preserved specimens are not acceptable for this staining technique.

1. Smear 1 to 2 drops of concentrated specimen on each of two slides and allow them to air-dry. Do not make the smears too thick. (A wet smear should be thin enough so that a printed page can be read through it.)
2. Fix slides by placing them in absolute methanol for 1 minute.
3. Flood slides with Kinyoun carbolfuchsin and stain for 5 minutes.
4. Rinse briefly (3 to 5 seconds) with 50 percent ethanol.
5. Rinse thoroughly with water.
6. Decolorize with 1 percent sulfuric acid for 2 minutes or until no more color runs from the slide.
7. Rinse with water. Drain.
8. Counterstain with methylene blue for 1 minute.
9. Rinse with water and allow to air-dry.
10. Examine the slide using the low and high dry objective. Use oil immersion to observe internal detail.

Results and Report for Kinyoun Acid-fast Stain Procedure

1. The color range of *Cryptosporidium parvum* (4 to 6 μm) and *Isospora belli* (~25 × ~15 μm) oocysts is from pink to deep purple, and four *(C. parvum)* sporozoites or one *(I. belli)* sporoblast are visible within oocysts. The background color is blue.
2. Microsporidia spores (1 to 2 μm) may resemble small yeast or bacteria.

    NOTE: Monoclonal antibody techniques may be needed to confirm the identity of light infections with *C. parvum.*

3. Cyanobacteriumlike bodies (CLB), also known as coccidian bodies *(Cyclospora),* appear as homogeneous pink to red spheres (8 to 10 μm).

    NOTE: These organisms have been found to cause severe diarrhea in immunocompetent patients as well as in patients with AIDS. Recent studies have tentatively placed these organisms in the genus *Cyclospora.*

4. Any parasites detected are reported by their scientific name, including both the genus and species names when possible.
5. Three specimens from alternate days should be examined.

Quality Control Considerations

1. Positive control slides should be made from 10 percent formalin-preserved *C. parvum* specimens. A positive control slide should be stained with each batch.

2. Check macroscopically to be sure the specimen adhered to the slide.
3. The ocular micrometer and microscope should be calibrated at least annually.
4. Quality control results should be recorded and the action plan for "out of control" results should be followed if needed.

BLOOD SMEAR PREPARATION AND STAINING FOR BLOOD PARASITES

These procedures are used for the recovery and identification of malaria, trypanosomes, microfilaria, *Babesia* spp., and *Leishmania donovani*. Both thin and thick smears should be prepared, stained, and examined. Thin smears offer the advantage of very little distortion of the parasite, but the disadvantage is that many fields must be examined to detect parasites when they are few in number. At least 200 to 300 thin film fields should be examined under oil immersion before reporting a negative smear. Although thick smear preparations often distort the parasite's morphology, the chances of detecting parasites are improved. Because this technique concentrates blood, the same volume of blood can be screened about three times faster than that in a thin smear. If improperly made, however, thick smears are useless. Fresh or EDTA-preserved specimens are preferred. Slides made from capillary blood must be made from a free-flowing drop that is not squeezed out or contaminated with alcohol.

Smear Preparation

Thin smears are prepared by touching a clean, grease-free slide to a small drop of blood so that the drop is near one end of the slide. A second spreader slide is held on edge at a 30-degree angle on the slide holding the specimen and drawn back into the drop, allowing it is spread along the edge of the spreader slide (Diagram 7–6). Then, smoothly and rapidly, push the spreader slide forward so that the blood spreads out and trails in a flat sheet. The amount of blood should be small enough so that it is all spread before the spreader reaches the end of the specimen slide. Allow to air-dry and stain as described. Screen the thin film for 30 minutes under 100× and also examine 100 to 200 microscopic fields of the thick film under oil immersion before reporting a specimen as negative.

Thick smears are prepared by touching a clean slide to a drop of blood. Using a corner of another slide, spread the blood evenly in a circular film about 15 mm in diameter. Allow to air-dry overnight, and lake the blood by placing the slide in distilled water. (Laking may be omitted if a 1:50 Giemsa stain is used). Laking causes RBCs to break open (i.e., lyse), causing hemoglobin's red color to disappear from the blood spot. Stain the laked blood smear according to the description that follows. Thin and thick

DIAGRAM 7–6

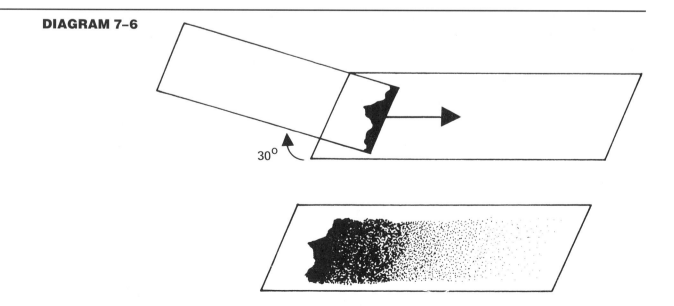

30°

smears can be made at opposite ends of the same slide. Fix only the thin smear prior to staining.

If filariasis is suspected, draw both diurnal and nocturnal blood samples to account for the periodicity of microfilaria. Perform a concentration test as described. In suspected malaria, if the first specimens are negative, retest the patient's blood every 6 to 8 hours for at least 3 days to account for the periodicity of schizogony. Unstained and stained blood smears should be stored protected from insects and light in slide storage boxes. Quality control known positive and negative slides should be used routinely for all staining procedures on blood and feces. Universal Precautions should be used at all times when handling blood or other body fluids.

Giemsa Staining Procedure

Thin smears: Fix the blood smear by immersing it in absolute methyl alcohol for 30 seconds. Place in working Giemsa stain (made by diluting stock Giemsa* 1:100 with pH 7.0 working buffer*) for 2 hours. The time may be reduced to 45 minutes if a 1:50 dilution is used or to 20 minutes if a 1:20 dilution is used. Rinse gently in buffer, drain, and air-dry. **(Do not blot.)** Examine under oil immersion as described previously.

Thick smears: Place unlaked smears in a 1:50 dilution of stock Giemsa for 45 minutes. (Do not use a 1:20 dilution.) Wash gently with buffer for 2 minutes. Excessive washing decolorizes the film. Air-dry and examine under oil immersion.

(*Note:* 3-minute quick stains for blood smears are available. Each laboratory should carefully compare results with standard staining methods.)

Results and Report for Giemsa Staining Procedure

1. To detect stippling, smears should be prepared within 1 hour after specimens are drawn.
2. Malaria, *Babesia* spp., trypanosomes, and leishmania cytoplasm stains blue, with nuclear material staining red. Schüffner's dots stain red. A microfilaria sheath may not stain, but the nuclei in the organism stain blue to purple.
3. Red cells stain pale red; WBCs, purple; eosinophilic granules, bright purple-red; and neutrophilic granules, deep pink-purple.
4. Any detected parasites are reported by their scientific name, including both the genus and species names when possible.

Quality Control Considerations

1. Because Giemsa stains are quite stable, it is usually necessary to check each new batch of stain only. If staining is done very infrequently, it is advisable that periodic checks be done, at least monthly.
2. The stain should be filtered if sediment appears on blood films. Known negative slides should be processed with each set of unknowns. If positive blood specimens are available from patients or quality control survey samples, control slides may be made and preserved by dipping them in absolute methanol. Check white blood cells and known parasites for color.
3. The ocular micrometer and microscope should be calibrated at least annually.
4. Quality control results should be recorded and the action plan for ''out of control'' results should be followed if needed.

KNOTT TECHNIQUE FOR CONCENTRATING MICROFILARIAE

When filariasis is suspected, it may be useful to concentrate blood in order to increase the possibility of finding microfilariae.

Procedure. The process should proceed as follows:

1. Obtain 2 mL of whole blood by venipuncture and immediately place it in a centrifuge tube containing 10 mL of 2 percent formalin.
2. Stopper the tube and mix thoroughly by inverting and shaking the tube. The formalin lakes red blood cells, fixes blood protozoa, and kills and straightens the bodies of microfilariae.

3. Centrifuge the tube for 5 minutes at 500*g* (1000 rpm) or let it stand stoppered overnight in the refrigerator.
4. Decant the supernatant.
5. Remove the sediment with a Pasteur pipette and spread in a thick film on a slide.
6. The sediment may be examined wet for microfilariae, or the slide may be allowed to dry overnight, followed by staining with Giemsa for 45 minutes. (See thick smear staining procedure described previously.) Destain in water (pH 7.2) for 10 to 15 minutes, allow to dry, and examine.

Of Note
1. Although not routinely performed, it may be useful to examine fresh blood when trypanosomes or microfilariae are suspected. To perform this technique, place a drop of fresh blood on a slide, add a coverslip to prevent clotting, and examine under low power (10×) for microfilariae or high dry power (40×) for trypanosomes. Especially when parasites are few in number, they may be detected by their characteristic motility. The undulating motion of the trypanosome and the whiplike motion of the microfilariae are easily spotted because they cause movement of surrounding red blood cells and thus may shorten the examination time needed for a positive diagnosis.
2. Other concentration techniques are available, including filtering laked blood through a fine-pore filter and then staining the filter for microfilariae, or passing blood through Sephadex filters, which selectively attach trypanosomes that can be later eluted. Stained blood films still must be examined to correctly identify the species of parasite.

STOLL EGG-COUNTING TECHNIQUE

After a parasite has been identified, it may be necessary to determine the intensity of the infection. Parasitic disease pathology usually correlates with the number of worms present, particularly for *Ascaris*, *Trichuris*, and hookworm disease. Daily egg outputs of these helminth species are known. Estimates of the worm burdens are accomplished by counting the number of eggs found in a known amount of feces and calculating the number of worms required to produce that many eggs. Many variables, such as diet, faulty digestion, cycles of egg production, and the consistency of the stool, influence the results, but counts performed before and during treatment may guide the course of therapy, and those done afterward will monitor its success. The best results are achieved when counts are done on succeeding specimens obtained over a period of several days so that the average daily egg output may be determined.

Procedure. The following steps should be followed:

1. Fill a 100-mL graduated cylinder to the 56-mL mark with 0.1 N sodium hydroxide.
2. Using applicator sticks, add enough feces to raise the fluid level to the 60-mL mark.
3. Add 10 small glass beads, stopper tightly, and shake until the feces are completely broken up. Hard stools may have to sit in the NaOH for several hours or overnight in the refrigerator to become soft.
4. When the feces are completely dissolved, shake the cylinder vigorously for 1 minute and immediately remove 0.075 mL of suspension and place it on a glass slide 1½ × 3 inches. Add a 22-mm square cover glass.
5. Use 100× magnification and count all eggs in the entire preparation. Be sure to look for eggs in any liquid around the edge of the cover glass.
6. Perform two counts using separate aliquots of 0.075 mL of suspension (total = 0.15 mL).

Calculation. The following steps should be taken:

1. The original fecal dilution is 1:15 (4 mL/60 mL). Because eggs in a total volume of 0.15 mL were counted, the total number of eggs in 1 mL of feces is found by multiplying the total count by 100 ($\frac{1}{15} \times 0.15 \times 100 = 1$).

2. Assuming that the average person passes 100 g of feces per day, it is possible to calculate the number of eggs per day by multiplying the answer by 100 (i.e., the original suspension total by 10,000).

3. To determine the number of female worms present, divide the number of eggs present in feces per day by the average number of eggs produced by one female per day.

   Female *Necator* spp.—7000 eggs/day
   Female *Ascaris* spp.—200,000 eggs/day
   Female *Trichuris* spp.—7500 eggs/day

4. Total worm burden is found by multiplying the answer found in Step 3 by two, because it is assumed that random infections provide one male worm for every female worm.

5. Some workers believe that correction factors for stool consistency must be used to obtain accurate results. To do this, the number obtained in Step 1 should be multiplied by the appropriate factor: formed stools = 1, mushy-formed = 1.5, mushy = 2, mushy-diarrheic = 3, flowing diarrheic = 4, and watery = 5.

Of Note

1. A more accurate count may be obtained if a 24-hour stool collection is saved and weighed. Exactly 4 g of mixed feces is then used in Step 1 of the counting procedure.

2. The calculation in Step 1 then is reported as eggs/gram of feces. This result may be multiplied by the total gram weight of the 24-hour specimen to give the total egg count/24 hours.

3. Clinically significant egg counts are as follows:

   a. *Necator* spp.—3000 to 12,000 eggs/gram of feces indicate the presence of about 70 to 350 worms and is associated with moderate, clinically significant infections.

   b. *Ancylostoma* spp.—6000 to 15,000 eggs/gram of feces indicate the presence of about 70 to 350 worms, because this parasite produces about twice as many eggs/day as *Necator* spp.

   c. *Ascaris* spp.—more than 16,000 eggs/gram of feces indicate the presence of at least 16 worms. Although infections of fewer than about 12 worms are usually asymptomatic, even one worm may cause clinical symptoms if, for example, it invades the bile duct.

   d. *Trichuris* spp.—300,000 eggs/gram of feces indicate the presence of about 600 worms and are associated with symptomatic infections. Fewer than 10,000 eggs/gram of feces are associated with asymptomatic infections.

PROTOZOA CULTURE MEDIA

Routine diagnosis of protozoan infections is usually possible without using culture methods, and few clinical labs offer culture techniques; however, several media are available that support growth of many protozoan species. Commonly used media for intestinal protozoa are either a semisolid base set up as slant tubes with a liquid overlay (Boeck and Drbohlav, Cleveland and Collier,[†] and McQuay diphasic charcoal medium) or a nutritive fluid (Balamuth). The axenic culture medium of Diamond is a useful diphasic medium in which a chick embryo extract is used as a liquid overlay for a slanted nutrient agar base. Diamond medium is primarily used in research centers and is most useful when stock cultures of *Entamoeba histolytica* must be maintained. Details for the in-house preparation of these basic media may be found in the references cited in this chapter.

Regardless of the medium chosen, careful handling of the culture is important to obtain successful results. Only fresh fecal specimens (less than 6 hours old) should be used, and at least two wet mounts made from the sediment should be examined after incubation, inasmuch as growth is slow and numbers may be few.

[†]Available as Bacto Entamoeba Medium, Difco Laboratories, Detroit, Michigan.

Procedure. Use the following steps:

1. To any of the prepared media listed previously, add a 5 mm loop of sterile rice powder.[‡]
2. Add about 1.5 mL of fluid or semifluid feces to each tube that is used; if the stool is formed, add a pea-sized portion to the tube and mix gently.
3. Incubate at 37°C for 24 hours; examine at least 0.1 mL of the surface of the semisolid sediment for trophozoites. PVA-fixed smears may be made from the surface material and stained with trichrome if desired.
4. All cultures not showing trophozoites should be transferred to new media by transferring the top half of the sediment to a tube containing fresh media. The new tube is then incubated at 37°C for 24 hours, after which the culture surface is examined as in Step 3. No further transfers are needed. The culture is considered negative at this point if parasites are not recovered.
5. To culture leishmania and *Trypanosoma cruzi*, use Novy-MacNeal-Nicolle (NNN)* medium at room temperature. Thirty percent defibrinated rabbit blood in the agar and antibiotics in the fluid overlay are preferred. Aspirated material, bone marrow, chancre, or blood may be used as culture specimens. Check condensate at the bottom of the slant for the presence of organisms for 1 month.

SEROLOGIC METHODS

With few notable exceptions such as tuberculosis, leprosy, and spirochetal diseases, microbial and viral infections are usually handled by the host in a relatively timely and straightforward manner. By contrast, the host's response to parasitic disease is much more complex and time-consuming. Elaborate life cycles and complex, changing antigenic structures create complex response problems for the host. Parasitic infections are often chronic because the host is rarely able to eliminate the source of infection, which forces the immune system to remain responsive. Various parasitic antigens have been shown to lead to immunosuppression, improper processing of antibody-antigen complexes by macrophages, disruption of normal B- and T-lymphocyte functions, and hypersensitivity responses. Immune complexes may form, leading to problems such as the autoimmune anemia or intravascular coagulation seen in American trypanosomiasis (Chagas' disease). All of these complicated mechanisms either cause or enhance the pathology seen in parasitic diseases.

All parasites elicit immune responses inducing the formation of IgM, IgG, and IgA antibodies. The entire range of immunologic responses is seen in parasitic diseases. Many protozoan parasites are effectively reduced or eliminated by macrophages that have become activated by sensitized T cells.

High levels of IgE antibody are frequently found in helminth infections. The IgE binds to mast cells, basophils, and eosinophils, causing the release of chemotactic factors, histamine activators, prostaglandins, and other mediators that produce the various hypersensitivity reactions. Infections caused by small parasites such as protozoa often induce delayed hypersensitivity responses, whereas helminth infections frequently induce T-cell–dependent eosinophilia and increased levels of IgE. Reactions including immediate hypersensitivity, anaphylaxis, and delayed hypersensitivity may be related to metabolic byproducts, surface antigens, or other substances released by the parasite.

During the tissue migration phase of helminths, the host responds to the infection by producing protective antibodies against the larval form. These antibodies provide resistance to reinfection by new larvae, resulting in a condition called concomitant immunity; this means that the host harbors the adult and is at the same time resistant to reinfection by the larval stage of the same parasite.

[‡]Available from Difco Laboratories, Detroit, Michigan.

The parasite's large size creates problems for the immune system. A helminth is too large to be completely destroyed by antibody mechanisms or by cellular responses, as are bacteria. It appears that a common mechanism for destroying these parasites requires that the surface of the adult be coated with antibody, which in turn attracts and binds white cells that release enzymes that damage the outer surface membrane of the parasite. Later, after the initial damage has been done, macrophages may become involved. In intestinal helminth infections in which adults are spontaneously eliminated, the level of IgE antibody often increases. It has been proposed that expulsion of adult worms results from a localized anaphylactic reaction mediated by the antibody and substances released by eosinophils. Others believe that intestinal goblet cells are stimulated by lymphokines released by activated T cells to secrete mucus that coats the damaged worm. This action, coupled with mast cell activation, increases gut motility to expel the parasite.

Although antibodies are often detectable in serum and may be useful guides when diagnosing diseases caused by parasites, they have little or no correlation with the course or prognosis of the disease. Later protection from reinfection by the parasite cannot be predicted based on circulating antibody levels. Clinical manifestations of parasitic diseases such as amebiasis of the liver, echinococcosis, trichinellosis, toxoplasmosis, and schistosomiasis are not always clear-cut, and when the measurable antibody titer reaches a detectable level in serum, it is often possible to confirm the diagnosis of these diseases serologically. Serology can also help identify a parasite's presence when it is in organs or other deep tissue sites such as the brain or muscle and no stages are recoverable in blood, urine, or feces.

Serologic testing is becoming more useful, particularly as commercial products become more readily available. Current methods fall into two general groups. One group includes procedures that directly combine with a parasite or its soluble antigen. For example, *Cryptosporidium parvum*, *Giardia lamblia*, and *Trichomonas vaginalis* can also be identified in clinical specimens by immunologic procedures. Indirect immunofluorescent (IIF), enzyme immunoassay (EIA), and enzyme-linked immunosorbent assay (ELISA) reagent test kits are available to test for these organisms. The IIF methods use monoclonal antibody against the parasite's cell wall and a fluorescein isothiocyanate-labeled anti-immunoglobulin to visualize the initial antibody-parasite complex. The ELISA methods capture organisms or soluble antigen by adding specimen samples to antibody-coated wells. Subsequent reactions cause a chromogen to change color to indicate the presence of bound antigen. New diagnostic procedures can be expected in the future, especially as DNA probe technology develops, but these tests will remain expensive for some time. In underdeveloped countries in which parasitic infections are common, high cost will limit the benefits from these procedures.

The second group of serology tests includes the many different methods used to recover and measure levels of circulating antibodies. Current methods include immunofluorescent antibody tests; slide, tube, and agar precipitin tests; complement fixation; particle agglutination tests; and enzyme-linked immunoassays, among others.

In the United States, serum for such studies is commonly sent for serologic testing to a State Public Health Reference Laboratory or to the Centers for Disease Control and Prevention (CDC) in Atlanta. Samples for CDC processing must be sent via state laboratories because CDC does not accept specimens sent directly by private laboratories or physicians. Most serum specimens may be shipped frozen or preserved with thimerosal (1:10,000 final concentration). The vial, containing at least 2 mL of serum, should indicate the preservative used. Table 7–1 lists the types of tests that are available generally for parasitic disease, as well as those tests performed at CDC. For state public health testing, consult locally. For more specific details about test procedures, the reader should consult the references at the end of this chapter.

At this time, several companies offer reagents and supplies for individual laboratories that want to perform their own procedures. Table 7–2 (page 141) includes procedures available from commercial suppliers. The list is not inclusive and in no way constitutes

Table 7–1. IMMUNODIAGNOSTIC TESTS FOR THE DIAGNOSIS OF PARASITIC DISEASES

Disease	Antibody Tests*	Antigen Tests	CDC Tests[†]
Acanthamoeba spp.	. . . . .	. . . . .	Culture[‡]
Amebiasis	EIA, IHA	No	IHA
Amebic meningoencephalitis	. . . . .	. . . . .	Culture[‡]
Babesiasis	IIF	No	IIF
Chagas' disease	EIA, IIF, CF	No	CF, IIF
Cryptosporidiosis	. . . . .	Yes	Confirm ID only
Cysticercosis	IB, EIA	No	IB
Echinococcosis	EIA, IHA, IB	No	IHA, IB
Fascioliasis	EIA	No	None
Filariasis	EIA	No	Confirm ID only
Giardiasis	. . . . .	Yes	Confirm ID only
Leishmaniasis	IIF, CF	No	CF, IIF
Malaria	IIF	No	IIF
Microsporidiosis	. . . . .	. . . . .	Culture[‡]
Naegleria spp	. . . . .	. . . . .	Culture[‡]
Paragonimiasis	EIA, IB	No	IB
Pneumocystosis	. . . . .	Yes	None
Schistosomiasis	EIA, IB	No	EIA, IB
Strongyloidiasis	EIA	No	EIA
Toxocariasis	EIA	No	EIA
Toxoplasmosis	EIA, IIF, EIA-IgM	No	IIF, EIA
Trichinellosis	BF, EIA	No	BF, EIA
Trichomoniasis	. . . . .	Yes	None
Trypanosoma cruzi	EIA, IIF, CF	No	CF, IIF

*EIA = enzyme immunoassay; IHA = indirect hemagglutination; IIF = indirect immunofluorescence; CF = complement fixation; IB = immunoblot; BF = bentonite flocculation; IgM = immunoglobulin M.

[†]The Division of Parasitic Diseases (DPD) at CDC provides confirmation of diagnoses when deemed essential by a state laboratory and DPD, especially for a potentially life-threatening infection. (Request the *Reference and Disease Surveillance* document for further information, from Centers for Disease Control and Prevention (CDC) in Atlanta, GA 30333.)

[‡]The Division of Parasitic Diseases (DPD) at CDC also cultures some parasites but only when prior arrangements have been made.

an endorsement by the authors of any product or supplier. It is merely a resource guide for those interested in parasitic serology.

Errors in serologic diagnosis may be related to mixed infections, cross-reacting antigens shared with other parasites or other microorganisms, or even to nonparasite-related diseases, as well as to errors in technique. Positive serology test results do not preclude previous infections, as responses are often long-lasting. Quality control tests using known positive and negative sera should always be performed. Direct detection methods require that known positive antigens or organisms for controls be tested as well.

Table 7–2. COMMERCIAL SEROLOGY KITS

Parasitic Disease	Test System	Supplier
Cryptosporidium	Enzyme immunoassay-plate	1, 3, 10
	Direct immunofluorescence assay	7
Entamoeba histolytica	Enzyme immunoassay	4
Giardia lamblia	Enzyme immunoassay-plate	1, 2, 3, 10
	Direct immunofluorescence assay	2, 7
Pneumocystis carinii	Enzyme immunoassay-slide	3
	Direct immunofluorescence assay	6, 7, 8
Toxoplasma gondii	Indirect hemagglutination	11
Trichinella spiralis	Latex agglutination	5, 11
Trichomonas vaginalis	Direct immunofluorescence	9

1. Alexon, Inc, 2319 Charleston Rd, Mountain View, CA 94043
2. Antibodies Inc, PO Box 1560, Davis, CA 95617
3. Dako Corp, 6392 Via Real, Carpinteria, CA 93013
4. Diamedix Corp, 2140 North Miami Way, Miami, FL 33127
5. Difco Laboratories, PO Box 1058A, Detroit, MI 38232
6. Disease Detection International, Inc, Irvine, CA (800-400-4334)
7. Meridian Diagnostics, Inc, 3741 River Hills Dr, Cincinnati, OH 45244
8. Sanofi Diagnostics Pasteur, 1000 Lake Hazeltine Dr, Chaska, MN 55218
9. SCIMEDX Corp, 400 Ford road, Denville, NJ 07834
10. Seradyn, Inc, Indianapolis, IN (800-345-0915)
11. Wampole Laboratories, Cranbury, NJ 08512

REAGENT PREPARATION

D'Antoni Iodine Stain

1. Use when preparing wet-mount preparations of fresh or concentrated feces.
2. Reagents:
   a. 1 g potassium iodine.
   b. 1.5 g powdered iodine crystals.
   c. Add reagents to 100 mL of distilled water and shake it well. Store in brown stoppered bottles; filter daily.

Polyvinyl Alcohol (PVA) Fixative

1. Use to preserve feces for transport or staining.
2. Reagents[§]:

a. Ethyl alcohol, 95 percent	156 mL
b. Mercuric chloride, aqueous (saturated)	312 mL
c. Glacial acetic acid	25 mL
d. PVA powder	20 mL
e. Glycerol	7.5 mL

   f. Mercuric chloride is prepared by dissolving 130 to 140 g of the salt in 1000 mL of distilled water. Heat to dissolve, then cool, filter, and store in a stock bottle.
   g. Add the PVA powder to the alcohol slowly, stirring. Heat to 75°C and stir until the solution is clear. Add the other reagents and allow to cool. Store in a closed container and use as needed. Decant the solution without disturbing the sediment.
3. Between 2 and 3 mL feces per 8 to 10 mL PVA solution is adequate for transport. (Check government regulations on mailing.) Slides may be made from the transport vial. Polyvinyl alcohol also can be used by mixing one drop of fluid stool in three drops of PVA solution on a slide and allowing it to dry overnight at 37°C before staining.

10 Percent Formalin

1. Use with the formalin-ethyl acetate sedimentation concentration method.
2. Reagents:

a. Formaldehyde	1 part
b. Physiologic saline	9 parts

[§]Bulk and prepackaged reagents are available from Meridian Diagnostics, Inc., Cincinnati, Ohio.

Zinc Sulfate Solution

1. Use with the zinc sulfate flotation concentration method.
2. Reagents:
   a. 330 g zinc sulfate (reagent grade).
   b. Distilled water (final volume—1 liter).
   c. Add reagent to the water with heat and stirring, and adjust the specific gravity to between 1.18 and 1.20, using a hydrometer.

Giemsa Stain

1. Use to stain blood parasites.
2. Reagents:
   a. Giemsa stain may be purchased as a concentrated stock or stock Giemsa can be prepared as follows:
      (1) Powdered Giemsa   1 g
      (2) Glycerol   66 mL
      (3) Methanol (absolute)   66 mL
   b. Grind the stain in a mortar containing 5 to 10 mL glycerol. Add the remaining glycerol and heat to 55°C in a water bath until the stain is dissolved. Cool and add the methanol. Let stand for 2 to 3 weeks. Filter and store in a brown bottle away from light.
3. Before use, dilute with Giemsa buffer.

Giemsa Buffer

1. Use with stock Geimsa stain.
2. Reagents:
   a. 0.067 M Na_2HPO_4 (disodium phosphate). Add 9.5 g to 1000 mL of distilled water. This is stock buffer No. 1.
   b. 0.067 M $NaH_2PO_4 \cdot H_2O$ (monosodium phosphate). Add 9.2 g to 1000 mL of distilled water. This is stock buffer No. 2.
3. Working buffer, pH 7.0, is prepared from stock buffers weekly and filtered before use. To 900 mL distilled water, add 61.1 mL of stock buffer No. 1 and 38.9 mL of stock buffer No. 2.

Trichrome Stain

1. Used to stain fecal smears for intestinal protozoa.
2. Reagents:
   a. Schaudinn solution: Saturated aqueous mercuric chloride; 130 to 140 g of mercuric chloride is added to 1000 mL of distilled water. Heat to dissolve, then cool and filter into a stock bottle. Working solution is prepared by mixing two parts of mercuric chloride solution with one part of 95 percent ethanol before use. Discard after use.
   b. Alcohol solutions: Various solutions may be prepared by diluting the appropriate volume of absolute (100 percent) ethanol with distilled water (e.g., a 70 percent solution is made by adding 30 mL of water to 70 mL of absolute alcohol). All alcohol solutions should be prepared fresh daily.
   c. Trichrome stain:
chromotrope 2R	0.6 g
light green SF	0.15 g
fast green FCF	0.15 g
phosphotungstic acid	0.7 g
acetic acid (glacial)	1.0 mL
distilled water	100 mL

      Mix the dry components and add the acetic acid; allow to stand for 30 minutes, then add to water. The stain should be purple. Staining more than 14 smears daily tends to weaken the stain. Strength returns if the stain is exposed to air for 3 to 8 hours.

      Prepared trichrome stain, made by Remal, is available through major laboratory supply companies.
   d. Acid alcohol is prepared by adding 1 mL acetic acid to 99 mL 90 percent ethanol.

NNN Medium

1. Use to culture blood, aspirates, bone marrow, biopsy, or other tissue material for *Leishmania* spp. and *Trypanosoma cruzi*.
2. Mix and bring to boiling the following ingredients:
   a. Agar   14 g
   b. Sodium chloride   6 g
   c. Distilled water   900 mL
3. Distribute medium to test tubes and sterilize in the autoclave.
4. Cool medium to 48°C and to each tube add one-third of its volume of sterilized defibrinated rabbit blood.
5. Mix thoroughly by rotation and allow to cool in a slanted position. Cooling is best done in an ice bath, as rapid cooling promotes water condensation in the tube. Organisms develop most rapidly in the supernate at the bottom of the tube.
6. Check for sterility by incubating the medium overnight at 37°C.

Kinyoun Carbolfuchsin

1. Dissolve 4 g of basic fuchsin in 20 mL of 95 percent ethanol (solution A).
2. Dissolve 8 g of phenol crystals in 100 mL of distilled water (solution B).
3. Mix solutions A and B together. Store at room temperature. Stable 1 year.

1 Percent Sulfuric Acid

1. Add 1 mL of concentrated sulfuric acid to 99 mL of distilled water. Store at room temperature. Stable 1 year.

Löffler Alkaline Methylene Blue

1. Dissolve 0.3 g of methylene blue in 30 mL of 95 percent alcohol.
2. Add 100 mL of dilute (0.01 percent) potassium hydroxide. Store at room temperature. Stable 1 year.

You have now completed the section on Clinical Laboratory Procedures. After reviewing this material with the aid of your learning objectives, proceed to the post-test.

BIBLIOGRAPHY

Chandler, AC, and Read, CP: *Introduction to Parasitology*, ed 10. John Wiley & Sons, New York, 1961, pp 402, 433.

Chitwood, M, and Lichtenfels, JR: Parasitological review. Identification of parasitic metazoa in tissue sections. Exp Parasitol 32:407, 1972.

Diamond, LS: Axenic culture of *Entamoeba histolytica*. Science 134:336, 1961.

Difco Manual of Dehydrated Cultural Media and Reagents for Microbiological and Clinical Laboratory Procedures, ed 9. Difco Laboratories, Detroit, 1974.

Frankerl, S, Reitman, S, and Sonnenwirth, AC (eds): *Gradwohl's Clinical Laboratory Methods and Diagnosis*, ed 8. CV Mosby, St Louis, 1980.

Garcia, LS, and Ash, LR: *Diagnostic Parasitology*, ed 4. Mosby, St Louis, 1994.

Garcia, LS, and Bruckner, DA: *Diagnostic Medical Parasitology*. American Society for Microbiology, Washington, DC, 1993.

Garcia, LS, and Bruckner, DA: *Diagnostic Medical Parasitology*, ed 2. Elsevier Science Publishers, New York, 1994.

Guttierrez, Y: *Diagnostic Pathology of Parasitic Infections with Clinical Correlations*. Lea & Febiger, Philadelphia, 1990.

MacInnis, AJ, and Vogue, M: *Experiments and Techniques in Parasitology*. WH Freeman, San Francisco, 1970.

Melvin, DM, and Brooke, MM: *Laboratory Procedures for the Diagnosis of Intestinal Parasites*, ed 3. US Department of Health, Education and Welfare Publication (CDC)-75-82821, Atlanta, 1985.

Salfelder, K: *Atlas of Parasitic Pathology* (Current Histopathology Series, Vol 20). Kluwer Academic Publishers, Norwell, MA, 1992.

Wheatley, WB: A rapid staining procedure for intestinal amoebae and flagellates. Am J Clin Pathol 2:990–991, 1951.

Wyngaarden, LB, and Smith, LH: *Cecil Textbook of Medicine*, ed 19. WB Saunders, Philadelphia, 1992.

Young, KH, et al: Ethyl acetate as a substitute for diethyl ether in the formalin-ether sedimentation technique. J Clin Microbiol 10:852–853, 1979.

POST-TEST   Mark True (T) or False (F) for each of the following: **(2 points each)**

_____ 1. In general, six sequential fecal specimens should be examined for the presence of any intestinal parasites.

_____ 2. Liquid or soft stools should be examined within 1 hour because trophozoites die rapidly.

_____ 3. Formed stools need not be refrigerated because protozoa have already formed cysts.

_____ 4. Wet mounts should be made when bloody mucus is noted in a stool specimen.

_____ 5. A castor oil enema may be used if only helminths are suspected.

_____ 6. It is not necessary to examine the whole slide if eggs or cysts are noted within the first few fields examined.

_____ 7. A careful examination of a stained thin smear of blood reveals the presence of blood parasites.

Discussion questions: **(5 points each)**

8. How should the microscope's light be adjusted for successful microscopic examination of wet mounts and why?

9. When should a cellophane tape test be done and why?

10. Name two types of concentration methods, explain the principles, and write the procedure for each method.

11. What is the specific gravity of the solution used in the zinc-sulfate concentration method? How is it checked?

12. Which eggs are not easily recovered by flotation methods?

13. What is used to extract fats in the sedimentation method?

14. List the advantages and disadvantages of thin and thick smears for blood parasites.

15. How is blood laked in the preparation of thick blood smears?

16. List the expected staining reactions for protozoa, using trichrome stain.

17. Name three protozoal culture media. What additional material is added to the culture at the time of inoculation?

18. Working Giemsa buffer is prepared from two stock solutions. What are the salts in each solution? What is the pH of the working buffer?

19. Match the reagents with the chemical components given: **(2 points each)**

a. _____ iodine crystals

b. _____ mercuric chloride

c. _____ rice powder

d. _____ light green SF

e. _____ monosodium phosphate

f. _____ phosphotungstic acid

g. _____ sugar

h. _____ 10% formalin

i. _____ 70% alcohol

j. _____ ethyl acetate

1. PVA
2. D'Antoni stain
3. Giemsa stain
4. Trichrome stain
5. Schaudinn solution
6. Balamuth
7. sedimentation
8. flotation

Each multiple choice question is worth **2 points**.

20. *Cryptosporidium parvum* oocysts are best detected in fecal specimens using the:
    a. Gram stain
    b. Iodine stain
    c. Methenamine silver stain
    d. Modified Ziehl-Neelson acid-fast stain
    e. Trichrome stain

21. The formalin-ethyl acetate concentration method for feces is used to demonstrate:
    a. Formation of amebic pseudopodia
    b. Hatching larval forms
    c. Motility of helminth larvae
    d. Protozoan cysts and helminth eggs
    e. Trophozoites

22. Bronchovascular lavage is the specimen of choice when:
    a. AIDS patients are suspected of having *Pneumocystis* pneumonia.
    b. Immunocompromised patients are suspected of having disseminated strongyloidiasis.
    c. Children are suspected of having pulmonary paragonimiasis.
    d. Any patient is suspected of having both toxoplasmosis and crytosporidiosis.
    e. Any patient is suspected of having *Acanthamoeba* spp. infection.

23. One of the following parasite procedures can be considered an urgent procedure (stat). That procedure is a/an:
    a. Ova and parasite examination for giardiasis
    b. Culture for amebic keratitis
    c. Blood film for malaria
    d. Baermann concentration for strongyloidiasis
    e. None of these

24. The best test procedure for correctly identifying *Enterobius vermicularis* infections is the:
    a. Formalin-ethyl acetate concentration method
    b. Cellophane tape test
    c. Zinc sulfate flotation method
    d. Entero capsule
    e. Knott concentration

25. Ameba trophozoite motility is best observed using a(n):
    a. Iodine-stained wet mount
    b. Unstained saline wet mount
    c. Unstained zinc sulfate flotation preparation
    d. Concentrated wet mount
    e. Giemsa stain

CHAPTER 8

Control and Treatment of Parasitic Disease

Most lay persons believe that treating an infected individual controls the parasitic disease and that avoiding an infected individual prevents catching the infection. These people also generally accept the idea that good hygienic practices lessen or prevent infections. Such concepts in fact do lead to a lower incidence of many diseases but, as you will see, the actual control of parasitic diseases in nature is far more complicated than this.

In order to control parasitic diseases adequately, we must give consideration to the parasite's life cycle; the cultural beliefs, personal hygiene, and dietary habits of the host; as well as community affluence; education; sanitation; and medical practices. Further, local ecologic and biologic factors as well as the general health of local domestic and wild animals must enter the picture.

A parasite's life cycle may involve a single host with no free-living stages (such as *Enterobius*, which is very easily spread), whereas others have a very complex life cycle (such as *Clonorchis*) involving multiple hosts and parasite stages.

Control of pinworm infection, for example, relies heavily on preventing the contamination of bed linens by wearing nonporous close-fitting clothing to bed, by sterilizing sheets in boiling water, and by frequent vacuum cleaning of rugs and furniture. Also important is attention to details such as covering toothbrushes or other personal articles in order to guard against exposure to bathroom dust, which may carry airborne eggs. Sunlight (ultraviolet) kills the larvae, as does dry heat; however, many household and other toxic chemicals do not penetrate the shell. Lack of cooperation between the patient and family members may actually hamper control and treatment.

Parasites such as *Schistosoma* that require an invertebrate host may be controlled by interrupting the life cycle, that is, by destroying the snail host itself or by destroying the infective cercaria larvae released into the water from the snail host. An advantage offered by this type of life cycle is that control measures do not depend heavily upon the involvement and the cooperation of the local citizenry but may be handled independently by knowledgeable experts in cooperation with the government.

Ensuring safe water and limiting snail populations are the two most important and viable control measures for schistosomiasis. An example of such successful preventive management has occurred in Puerto Rico. Early in the control campaign, a trial mass chemotherapy treatment of infected individuals led to the death of some persons because of drug side effects. Chemotherapy was suspended and attention was focused on snail control. A molluscan competitor was introduced into ponds, lakes, and rivers in an effort to reduce the numbers of the specific host species. Concurrently, the project managers improved sanitary waste disposal systems, thus reducing the exposure of the snails to infective miracidium. By the mid-1960s, some 15 to 20 years of work began to show success. In most areas of Puerto Rico, the rate of infection in the population fell from 20 percent to almost zero.

Because schistosomiasis is still a major problem in many parts of the world, similar control methods are being tried elsewhere. However, another important control strategy is human behavior modification. Because human infection with schistosomiasis occurs when cercariae penetrate bare skin, something as simple as wearing wading boots in water can break the parasite's life cycle. Shoes serve the same purpose in preventing hookworm and *Strongyloides* infections. Most important, by teaching people to use toilets or latrines, infected urine or feces do not contaminate soil or water supplies.

In controlling the spread of other parasitic diseases, chemical measures have had varying degrees of success. Remember—dormant stages of parasites, such as eggs and cysts, are generally resistant to toxic substances, which makes control of the environment difficult. A practical solution in many cases is vector control when an arthropod is involved. For instance, sprays and dips reduce flea and tick infestations in livestock and domestic pets even though it does not clear the environment. Biodegradable chemicals in water supplies have been used to control black fly larvae, and insecticide sprays are widely used to control the tsetse fly vector of trypanosomiasis.

The World Health Organization (WHO) sponsored an ambitious program to eradicate malaria worldwide. Early in the program, investigating members of the project found many mosquitoes resting inside houses. Consequently, they had the inside walls of houses and other buildings sprayed with DDT. This initially aggressive attack dramatically reduced the malaria problem in parts of Africa, but when local follow-up procedures became lax because of initial success, the incidence of malaria climbed dramatically. Some observers have claimed that the WHO program contributed greatly to the DDT resistance seen in mosquitoes, but the resistance problem can actually be traced to indiscriminant agricultural use of the chemical.

Another problem hampered WHO's African mosquito attack. Either two insect groups existed (house-dwelling and bush-dwelling), or some of the house-dwelling mosquitoes changed their behavior patterns and became bush-dwelling mosquitoes. Some investigators believed that the DDT house-spraying measures may have selected for the bush-dwelling mosquitoes. However, when the spraying stopped, the house-dwelling mosquitoes reappeared, suggesting still another biologic change. Regardless of the reasons for the changes, the DDT experience offers an example of the importance of understanding the complex biology and behavior patterns of insect vectors when choosing control strategies.

Of serious ecologic concern, however, is the history of indiscriminant spraying of insecticide prior to human understanding of the biologic impact of chemicals such as DDT on all plants and animals in the food chain, as well as our failure to predict that such spraying would cause selection for insect vectors resistant to chemicals. These human errors should not be allowed to recur.

A more successful control experience occurred in Central America, where a well-planned strategy was used to control *Culicoides* spp., which bred in the Farfan Swamp in the Panama Canal Zone. These tiny biting gnats (no-see-ums) can fly through normal window screen mesh and forced workers caring for military communications equipment located in the swamp to wear finely meshed protective suits. Because temperatures often reached more than 90°F, the obvious discomforts forced other control measures to be sought. Chemical control of the insect in the swamp began in the early 1950s, but the gnat developed genetic resistance to the insecticide, making other control measures necessary.

The Farfan Swamp, although fed by a freshwater stream, was brackish because seawater backed into it. Because the endemic *Culicoides* spp. breeds only in salty water, tidal gates were built to keep the sea water out of the swamp. Gradually, the swamp's water became fresh, and by the late 1950s, the gnat population had diminished to an acceptable level. Later, in the mid-1960s, a canal dredging operation began dumping its dredge into the swamp, causing the water to become salty again. This change caused the gnat population to grow, and efforts were then made to halt dumping in the Farfan Swamp. It took about two years to clear the salt once again from the swamp water, and consequently, to bring the *Culicoides* back under control.

Various other methods of biologic insect and parasitic control have been tried. Elimination of primary screwworm fly myiasis from the southeastern United States was accomplished by releasing numerous male *Cochliomyia (Callitroga) hominivorax* flies that had been sterilized by irradiation. Competitive mating decreased the offspring to below critical mass levels for breeding. Similar successful elimination in the southwestern United States has not been achieved because the insect population entering from Mexico could not be adequately controlled at the same time. By contrast, the Florida peninsula effectively isolated its area from invading flies. More recently, the state of California used irradiated flies in its campaign against the Mediterranean fruit fly. Daily, 20,000 irradiated flies raised in an agricultural research station in Hawaii were shipped to California. This helped save the fruit crop and lessened the need for chemical control measures. This example illustrates that combining various strategies can control insect populations.

Serious efforts are also being expended on perfecting other control systems. Immunization has already proved successful against several serious parasites of domestic animals. Other biologic methods are also being explored, such as improved insect traps using pheromones; genetic manipulation of insect hosts; introduction of predators for insect, snail, and other host species; introduction of competitive species of nonpathogenic parasites or nonsupportive hosts; and mass treatment of host populations with chemotherapeutic agents. For example, India, which spends 45 percent of its national health budget controlling malaria, is now looking to alternatives to the millions of dollars spent on pesticides. These include breeding fish in waters that harbor mosquito larvae and later selling the fish, filling in pits and creating usable land, and planting eucalyptus trees in swamps to soak up water and later using the wood for cooking and construction.

Cultural behavior of world populations both aids and hinders the control of parasitic diseases. For instance, the dietary customs of Jewish and Moslem peoples have greatly reduced their exposure to *Taenia solium* and *Trichinella spiralis* infections. Then again, people in many parts of the world, including the United States, still use untreated human waste (known as night soil) to fertilize crops. They also bathe and wash clothes and cooking utensils in water contaminated with human waste. Such behavior obviously promotes the transmission of parasites. In some wealthy countries, again including the United States, many people are getting back to nature or vacationing in health resorts offering natural or untreated water and foods. Unfortunately, one side effect to this lifestyle has been some increase in giardiasis as well as exposure to other amebic diseases. Nevertheless, affluence has many benefits. Home freezers contribute to the control of trichinosis, because freezing pork for 6 days at 20°F kills encysted larvae. Similarly, freezing foodstuffs for various time periods can prevent other diseases. In addition, use of window screens in more affluent countries is greatly reducing human exposure to disease-carrying vectors. The most valuable invention, however, for preventing the spread of parasitic infections has been the flush toilet, and its use everywhere is accompanied by decrease in disease. Probably the most effective control measure among our variety of measures may also be the hardest one to accomplish—the changing of human behavior through education and demonstrated rewards of improved health. The WHO campaign to teach people in endemic areas to strain drinking water through tee shirt cotton is successfully reducing the incidence of *Dracunculus* infections.

From the foregoing, it is evident that, on paper at least, parasitic diseases can be controlled by various methods, but until widespread control is achieved, a need continues for chemotherapeutic intervention for infected individuals. Before treating a given infection with chemotherapy, the physician weighs several factors, including the severity and duration of infection, the health conditions of the host, and the availability and toxicity of the drug treatment. If the toxicity or side effects of a treatment are more hazardous to the patient than the disease itself, then treatment may be reasonably withheld. Furthermore, if the chance of reinfection is great and the disease is mild, then treatment is probably questionable at best.

Once the decision to treat an infection has been made, consideration of the need to treat asymptomatic family members or others closely associated with the infected individual is important. For example, some parasites such as *Giardia* may be easily spread to others in a family or in an institutional setting, so treatment of other resident individuals may indeed be appropriate. Because *Trichomonas vaginalis* is transmitted sexually, all partners of the infected person should be treated as well. It is useless to treat others or isolate an infected person if direct transmission is not possible. This is why it is important to understand life cycles.

Some parasitic infections need not be treated because they are at a stage of low worm burdens, are self-limiting and nonpathogenic, and probably will not be transmitted to others. Some infections, however, require chemotherapy and/or surgical intervention. Cysticercosis and hydatid cysts at present require surgery, but treatment of amebiasis of the liver or appendix less often requires surgical attention, because more effective chemotherapeutics are now available. Promising new drugs are under study.

The objectives of a treatment program should be to stop the parasite's growth and reproduction, to kill parasites without inducing a harmful host response, and/or to expel parasites from the host. Finding those drugs that are selective for parasitic metabolic systems without adversely affecting human systems has been difficult. Not surprisingly, many drugs are rather toxic, especially the ones that affect energy metabolism. A variety of drugs currently in use are known carcinogens or teratogens.

Most drugs commonly used to treat infections affect various metabolic pathways such as energy metabolism, cell wall synthesis, protein synthesis, membrane function, nucleic acid synthesis, or cofactor synthesis. Several drugs affect neuromuscular systems of the helminths. The selective action of many antiprotozoal drugs results from either preferential absorption of the drug by the parasite or from the ability of the drug to discriminate between isofunctional targets in the host cells versus those in the parasitic cell. Little is known about the selective action of most antihelminthic chemicals.

Drug resistance develops when pathogenic organisms are able to metabolize the drug to an inactive form, to alter their permeability to the drug, to use a metabolic pathway not affected by the drug, to increase enzyme production in order to overcome the level of the drug being administered, or to change the drug's binding site target on or inside the organism.

The extent to which each of the drug resistance factors mentioned affects the treatment of parasitic disease is not fully known. Alterations in permeability, drug-binding activity, and enzyme production all have been demonstrated for some parasites, with altered permeability being the single most common resistance mechanism. Changes with respect to binding activity and enzyme production can be genetically passed to offspring.

Table 8–1 (page 152) contains a partial listing of chemotherapeutic agents commonly in use, along with some of their important side effects. The reader will find a further listing and updating of agents and side effects in the *Medical Letters* cited in the bibliography for this chapter.

Treatment of amebiasis caused by *Entamoeba histolytica* (see Item 11 on Table 8–1) depends upon the severity of the clinical symptoms and on the parasites' locations in the host. Debate over the treatment of asymptomatic carriers continues; however, when treated, the person is usually given diiodohydroxyquin or diloxanide furoate. When either mild or severe intestinal signs are evident, metronidazole plus diiodohydroxyquin is the treatment of choice. Extraintestinal amebiasis may be treated using metronidazole. Diiodohydroxyquin is also required with a concurrent bowel infection. Because newer drugs are less toxic, emetine is no longer considered the best treatment for extraintestinal amebiasis. However, the higher cost and limited availability of newer drugs in other parts of the world have perpetuated the use of emetine.

Infections with *Trichomonas vaginalis* in either sex are effectively treated with the oral medication metronidazole. This drug should not be taken by pregnant women, however. Topical preparations containing halogenated hydroxyquinolines are useful in relieving the symptoms of vaginitis but may not completely eliminate the parasite because the preparation may not reach every organism. Other topical preparations are also available. Sexual partners should be treated simultaneously.

The treatment of helminths relies on the correct identification of the parasite involved. Generally, mebendazole and pyrantel pamoate are considered the drugs of choice in the treatment of most intestinal nematode infections. Thiabendazole is useful against cutaneous and visceral larval migrans and *Strongyloides stercoralis*. Niclosamide is effective against cestodes. Praziquantel is effective against all *Schistosoma* spp. and other flukes, while metrifonate or oxamniquine are suitable alternates for some schistosomes.

Treatment of filariasis is accomplished with diethylcarbamazine; however, some authorities recommend excision of the adult *Onchocerca* worm before treatment because this drug does not kill the adult. An alternative treatment for onchocerciasis begins with a 3-week course of diethylcarbamazine followed by suramin. Suramin kills the adult worm. Further, antihistamines or corticosteroids may be needed to reduce the allergic (Mazzotti) reaction to disintegrating microfilariae. Extreme caution is needed while treating onchocerciasis, because the allergic reaction may be fatal.

Early diagnosis and treatment of African trypanosomiasis is important because treatment after the central nervous system is involved is quite difficult. Suramin sodium is the drug of choice early on, but because it does not cross the blood-brain barrier, melarsoprol is needed for the late disease stages. Nifurtimox is most useful when treating *Trypanosoma cruzi* infections. All drugs for African trypanosomiasis are very toxic, and most should be administered during hospitalization.

The treatment of malaria follows two strategies—clinical cure and radical cure. A clinical cure is accomplished when symptoms are relieved and asexual parasites are eliminated from peripheral circulation. However, this treatment does not necessarily mean that all parasites have been eradicated from the body. Chloroquine phosphate is the drug of choice for treating all species of malaria sensitive to the drug—it produces a clinical cure but does not completely eliminate the parasite from the host in those infections caused by relapsing species of malaria. A radical cure (elimination of secondary tissue schizonts) for *Plasmodium vivax* and *P. ovale* is accomplished using primaquine phosphate as the second course of treatment.

Travelers to endemic areas, including former residents who are returning after living in nonmalarious areas for some time, are advised to begin taking chloroquine phosphate (Aralen) once weekly 1 to 2 weeks prior to travel and to continue throughout their stay in the endemic area and for 4 weeks after return. In addition, primaquine phosphate should be taken for 2 weeks after leaving the area. This prophylactic course normally prevents disease. Because chloroquine phosphate does not prevent liver invasion by the parasite, it is especially important to use primaquine to prevent a relapse with *P. vivax* or *P. ovale*. Individuals deficient in glucose-6-phosphate dehydrogenase (G6PD) should not use primaquine.

Various strains of *P. falciparum* have become resistant to chloroquine. Successful treatment of these infections requires the use of alternative antimalarials such as a combination of pyrimethamine and sulfadoxine. Quinine may be used in place of chloroquine phosphate.

For prophylaxis, the Centers for Disease Control and Prevention recommends using mefloquine (Lariam) in place of chloroquine phosphate once weekly for travelers in endemic areas of resistant malaria. It should be noted that areas of chloroquine-resistant malaria are no longer limited to East Africa but now include many locations in Central Africa as well.

Since the discovery and later identification of the human immunodeficiency virus (HIV) and its relationship to AIDS and AIDS-related complex (ARC), several opportunistic parasitic infections have been recognized as important problems for immunocompromised patients. These problems are not limited only to AIDS patients but also affect individuals who have compromised immune systems due to congenital absence or abnormal development of the immune system, malignancy, irradiation, cytotoxic drug therapy, or other underlying infections. Aside from parasitic disease, these patients have higher incidence of bacterial, viral, and fungal infections as well.

There has been a high number of cases of parasitic infections reported in immunocompromised patients. The most likely patient population, continuing to grow in number, is the AIDS group consisting of IV drug users, homosexual and bisexual men, prostitutes, hemophiliacs, persons seeking treatment for sexually transmitted diseases, persons having multiple sexual partners, persons who consider themselves at risk, and children born to infected mothers.

AIDS is not curable at the present time, but it is generally preventable for adults.

Prevention is accomplished by avoiding high-risk practices such as unprotected sex and drug needle-sharing. All medical care workers must follow the Occupational Safety and Health Administration's (OSHA) rules related to bloodborne pathogens, referred to as the "Universal Precautions" with blood or other body fluids. These rules provide a way for medical personnel to avoid becoming infected with any disease-causing organism, not just HIV. If these practices are not followed, workers may become infected and may even infect fellow workers or others.

At least eight parasitic infections are most commonly reported in immunocompromised patients. Seven of these are protozoan and the other one is caused by *Strongyloides stercoralis*. Immunocompetent hosts may harbor *Strongyloides* for years without symptoms other than an unexplained eosinophilia. When the patient becomes compromised, the number of larvae and adults increases rapidly, producing disseminated strongyloidiasis. As *S. stercoralis* rhabditiform larvae become infective filariform larvae, they carry bacteria with them as they invade the intestinal mucosa; bacteremia, pneumonia, and even meningitis can result. *Strongyloides* hyperinfections have also been found in patients with leukemias, lymphomas, fungal infections, leprosy, tuberculosis, and other conditions such as renal disease and asthma. Patients who have high eosinophilia (10% to 50%) and unexplained bacteremia or other problems caused by enteric bacteria should be tested for strongyloidiasis.

The protozoa most commonly encountered in immunocompromised humans include: *Entamoeba histolytica, Giardia lamblia, Pneumocystis carinii* (pneumonia), *Toxoplasma gondii* (encephalitis), *Cryptosporidium parvum, Isospora belli*, and five genera of Microsporidia. The intestinal protozoa usually cause chronic diarrhea and chronic wasting syndrome ("slim disease"). Although *E. histolytica* and *G. lamblia* are not considered opportunistic parasites, they must be mentioned in this list because they can produce rather severe symptoms in immunocompromised hosts. Extraintestinal invasion by *E. histolytica* is more likely to occur in these patients as well.

Expectorated sputum, bronchoscopy specimen, or open-lung biopsy can be stained and evaluated for *Pneumocystis*. Treatment is a rather involved process because the patients frequently have adverse reactions to medications (trimethoprim-sulfamethoxazole or pentamidine isethionate).

Clinically active cases in both immunocompromised patients and diagnosed congenital disease should be treated. The standard treatment regimen consists of pyrimethamine and sulfadiazine. Also, lifelong maintenance therapy is frequently required.

Cryptosporidium is difficult to treat, requiring fluid replacement, nutrition, and antidiarrheal medication. Spiramycin and eflornithine have given limited success. *Isospora* infections are treated with trimethoprim-sulfamethoxazole for approximately 1 month.

Microsporidia have been found throughout the body, but the most frequent infection found in AIDS patients has been caused by *Enterocytozoon bieneusi*. These patients have chronic diarrhea, fever, and weight loss that mimic other intestinal infections. It is important to thoroughly investigate these symptoms because there is no satisfactory treatment for these parasites.

Treatment of parasitic diseases relies heavily on accurate diagnosis followed by good judgment on the part of the physician. Factors such as drug toxicity, the parasite's location in the host, the length of the treatment course, the method of the drug's administration, other drugs being administered, and the general condition of the patient must all be considered in order to provide maximum benefit. If only one drug is available, however, and the patient's condition necessitates treatment, there may be no other choice. Furthermore, certain long treatment schedules may facilitate parasitic resistance to the drug or create cumulative toxicity problems for the patient. Finally, good nutritional management and patient involvement in self-care is important to help the patient overcome infection and promote resistance to subsequent infections.

The CDC can provide detailed information about the treatment and use of various drugs as well as supply drugs for treating rare diseases. Note that some drugs are teratogenic in animals, and special care should be taken to avoid prescribing them to pregnant women. Teratogens are noted in Table 8–1, as are others that may have more severe effects for pregnant women or young children.

Table 8-1. CHEMOTHERAPY OF PARASITIC DISEASES

Infecting Organism	Disease	Chemotherapeutic Agent	Adverse Reactions*
Acanthamoeba spp.	Meningoencephalitis	Amphotericin B and sulfadiazine or sulfisoxazole	**Rash**, photosensitivity, hepatic and renal toxicity, blood dyscrasia, vasculitis
Ancylostoma braziliense	Cutaneous larval migrans; creeping eruption	Thiabendazole	**Nausea, vomiting, vertigo, rash**, leukopenia, color vision disturbance, tinnitus, shock
Ancylostoma duodenale	Hookworm	Mebendazole[†] or	**GI disturbance**
		Pyrantel pamoate	**GI disturbance**, dizziness, rash, fever
Ascaris lumbricoides	Roundworm	Mebendazole[†] or	**GI disturbance**
		Pyrantel pamoate	**GI disturbance**, dizziness, rash, fever
Balantidium coli	Balantidiasis	Tetracycline or	**Anorexia, nausea**, vomiting, renal and hepatic impairment
		Metronidazole[†]	**Nausea, headache**, vomiting, diarrhea, vertigo, insomnia, ataxia
Clonorchis sinensis	Chinese liver fluke	Praziquantel	Sedation, abdominal discomfort, fever, sweating, nausea, eosinophilia, photosensitivity, urticaria, vomiting, and diarrhea
Dientamoeba fragilis	Dientamoebiasis	Iodoquinol or	**Iodine toxicoderma**, rash, slight thyroid enlargement, nausea
		Tetracycline or	**Anorexia, nausea**, vomiting, renal and hepatic impairment
		Paromomycin	**GI disturbance**
Diphyllobothrium latum	Fish tapeworm	Niclosamide[†] or	Nausea, abdominal pain
		Praziquantel	Sedation, abdominal discomfort, fever, sweating, nausea, eosinophilia, photosensitivity, urticaria, abdominal pain, vomiting, and diarrhea
Dracunculus medinensis	Filariasis; guinea worm	1. Ivermectin[†]	**Allergic and febrile reactions** due to worm
		2. Niridazole or	**Immunosuppression**, vomiting, cramps, dizziness, headache
		Metronidazole[†] or	**Nausea, headache**, vomiting, diarrhea, vertigo, insomnia, ataxia
		Thiabendazole	**Nausea, vomiting, vertigo, rash**, leukopenia, color vision disturbance, tinnitus, shock
Echinococcus spp.	Hydatid cyst	Mebendazole[†] or Albendazole	**GI disturbance**
Entamoeba histolytica	Amebiasis	Iodoquinol or	**Iodine toxicoderma**, rash, slight thyroid enlargement, nausea
		Paromomycin	**GI disturbance**
	Intestinal disease	Metronidazole[†] plus	**Nausea, headache**, vomiting, diarrhea, vertigo, insomnia, ataxia
		Iodoquinol	**Iodine toxicoderma**, rash, slight thyroid enlargement, nausea
	Hepatic disease	Metronidazole[†] plus	**Nausea, headache**, vomiting, diarrhea, vertigo, insomnia, ataxia
		Iodoquinol	**Iodine toxicoderma**, rash, slight thyroid enlargement, nausea

	Table 8–1. CHEMOTHERAPY OF PARASITIC DISEASES (Continued)		
Infecting Organism	**Disease**	**Chemotherapeutic Agent**	**Adverse Reactions***
Enterobius vermicularis	Pinworm	Pyrantel pamoate or	**GI disturbance**, dizziness, rash, fever
		Mebendazole[†]	**GI disturbance**
Fasciola hepatica	Liver rot: sheep liver fluke	Bithionol or	Photosensitivity skin reaction, vomiting, diarrhea, abdominal pain, urticaria
		Praziquantel	Sedation, abdominal discomfort, fever, sweating, nausea, eosinophilia, photosensitivity, urticaria, abdominal pain, vomiting, and diarrhea
Fasciolopsis buski	Fascioliasis	Praziquantel or	Sedation, abdominal discomfort, fever, sweating, nausea, eosinophilia, photosensitivity, urticaria, abdominal pain, vomiting, and diarrhea
		Niclosamide[†] or	Nausea, abdominal pain
		Tetrachloroethylene	**Epigastric burning**, **dizziness**, **headache**
Giardia lamblia	Giardiasis	Quinacrine or	Vomiting, vertigo, headache, psychosis, blood dyscrasia, ocular damage, rash, hepatic necrosis
		Metronidazole[†]	**Nausea**, **headache**, **vomiting**, diarrhea, vertigo, insomnia, ataxia
Heterophyes heterophyes	Heterophyiasis, intestinal fluke	Praziquantel	Sedation, abdominal discomfort, fever, sweating, nausea, eosinophilia, photosensitivity, urticaria, abdominal pain, vomiting, and diarrhea
Hymenolepis nana	Dwarf tapeworm	Praziquantel	Sedation, abdominal discomfort, fever, sweating, nausea, eosinophilia, photosensitivity, urticaria, abdominal pain, vomiting, and diarrhea
Isospora belli	Intestinal disease	Trimethoprim-sulfamethoxazole (TMP-SMX) (teratogenic in animals)	Rash, photosensitivity, hepatic and renal toxicity, blood dyscrasia, vasculitis
Leishmania braziliensis complex or	Leishmaniasis: mucocutaneous	Antimony Na gluconate (stibogluconate sodium)	Muscle pain and joint stiffness, bradycardial colic, diarrhea, rash
L. mexicana complex			
L. donovani complex	Leishmaniasis: visceral	Antimony Na gluconate (stibogluconate sodium) or	Muscle pain and joint stiffness, bradycardial colic, diarrhea, rash
		Pentamidine isethionate	**Hypotension-hypoglycemia**, **vomiting**, **blood dyscrasias**, **renal damage**, rash, hepatic toxicity
L. tropica complex	Leishmaniasis: cutaneous	Antimony Na gluconate (stibogluconate sodium)	Muscle pain and joint stiffness, bradycardial colic, diarrhea, rash
Loa loa	Filariasis: eyeworm	Diethylcarbamazine or ivermectin[†]	**Allergic and febrile reactions** due to worm
Metagonimus yokogawai	Metagonimiasis: intestinal fluke	Praziquantel or	Sedation, abdominal discomfort, fever, sweating, nausea, eosinophilia, photosensitivity, urticaria, abdominal pain, vomiting, and diarrhea
		Tetrachloroethylene	**Epigastric burning**, **dizziness**, **headache**, drowsiness, Antabuse-like effect with alcohol

Table continued on following page

Table 8-1. CHEMOTHERAPY OF PARASITIC DISEASES (Continued)

Infecting Organism	Disease	Chemotherapeutic Agent	Adverse Reactions*
Microsporidium spp.	Tissue parasites	No effective treatment	
Naegleria fowleri	Primary meningoencephalitis	Amphotericin B	**Chills**, **sweating**, **fever**, **muscle pain**, **abdominal pain**, **nausea**, **vertigo**
Necator americanus	Hookworm	Mebendazole[†] or	**GI disturbance**
		Pyrantel pamoate	**GI disturbance**, headache, dizziness, rash, fever
Onchocerca volvulus	Filariasis; river blindness	1. Ivermectin[†]	**Allergic and febrile reactions** due to worm
		2. Diethylcarbamazine plus suramin[†]	**Rash**, **pruritus**, **paresthesias**, vomiting, peripheral neuropathy, shock
Opisthorchis viverrini	Opisthorchiasis: liver fluke	Praziquantel	Sedation, abdominal discomfort, fever, sweating, nausea, eosinophilia, photosensitivity, urticaria, abdominal pain, vomiting, and diarrhea
Paragonimus westermani	Paragonimiasis; lung fluke	Praziquantel or	Sedation, abdominal discomfort, fever, sweating, nausea, eosinophilia, photosensitivity, urticaria, abdominal pain, vomiting, and diarrhea
		Bithionol	Photosensitivity skin reaction, vomiting, diarrhea, abdominal pain, urticaria
Pediculus humanus var. *corporis* or *capitis*	Lice	1% permethrin or	Irritation to skin, eyes, and mucous membranes
		Pyrethrin with piperonyl butoxide or 0.5% malathion lotion or 1% lindane	Irritation to skin, eyes, mucous membranes; ragweed-sensitized persons should not use
Phthirus pubis	Crab lice	1% permethrin	Irritation to skin, eyes, and mucous membranes
Plasmodium falciparum	Malignant malaria (chloroquine-susceptible) (Note: Chemoprophylaxis: chloroquine phosophate or mefloquine)	Chloroquine phosphate (Note: no primaquine[†] after)	Headache, vomiting, confusion, skin eruptions, retinal injury
	(chloroquine-resistant)	Quinine sulfate and	**Cinchonism**, **hypotension**, **arrhythmias**, blood dyscrasia, photosensitivity, blindness
		Pyrimethamine plus	**Folic acid deficiency**, blood dyscrasia, rash, vomiting, convulsions, shock
		Sulfadiazine	**Rash**, photosensitivity, hepatic and renal toxicity, blood dyscrasia, vasculitis
	(comatose patient)	Quinine (parenteral)	**Cinchonism**, **hypotension**, **arrhythmias**, blood dyscrasia, photosensitivity, blindness
Plasmodium malariae	Quartan malaria	Chloroquine phosphate (Note: no primaquine[†] after infection)	Headache, vomiting, confusion, skin eruptions, retinal injury
Plasmodium ovale	Ovale malaria	Chloroquine phosphate	Headache, vomiting, confusion, skin eruptions, retinal injury
	(radical cure)	followed by primaquine[†] phosphate (prevents relapses)	**Hemolytic anemia** in G6PD deficient patients, neutropenia, nausea, hypertension; do not use during pregnancy

Table 8–1. CHEMOTHERAPY OF PARASITIC DISEASES (Continued)

Infecting Organism	Disease	Chemotherapeutic Agent	Adverse Reactions*
Plasmodium vivax	Tertian malaria	Chloroquine phosphate	Headache, vomiting, confusion, skin eruptions, retinal injury
	(radical cure)	followed by primaquine[†] phosphate (prevents relapses)	**Hemolytic anemia** in G6PD deficient patients, neutropenia, nausea, hypertension; do not use during pregnancy
Pneumocystis carinii	Pneumocystosis	Trimethoprim-sulfamethoxazole or	Rash, photosensitivity, hepatic and renal toxicity, blood dyscrasia, vasculitis
		Pentamidine isethionate	Breathlessness, dizziness, headache, tachycardia, vomiting, itching
Sarcoptes scabiei	Mites; scabies	5% permethrin	Irritation to skin, eyes, and mucous membranes
Schistosoma haematobium	Schistosomiasis; bladder worm	Praziquantel	Sedation, abdominal discomfort, fever sweating, nausea, eosinophilia
Schistosoma japonicum	Schistosomiasis; blood fluke	Praziquantel	Sedation, abdominal discomfort, fever, sweating, nausea, eosinophilia
Schistosoma mansoni	Schistosomiasis; blood fluke, swamp fever	Praziquantel or	Sedation, abdominal discomfort, fever, sweating, nausea, eosinophilia
		Oxamniquine (Vansil)	Headache, fever, dizziness, nausea, insomnia, diarrhea, hepatic enzyme changes
Strongyloides stercoralis	Threadworm	Thiabendazole	**Nausea, vomiting, vertigo, rash,** leukopenia, color vision disturbance, tinnitus, shock
Taenia saginata	Cestode; beef tapeworm	Niclosamide[†] or	Nausea, abdominal pain
		Praziquantel	Sedation, abdominal discomfort, fever, sweating, nausea, eosinophilia, photosensitivity, urticaria, abdominal pain, vomiting, and diarrhea
Taenia solium	Cestode; pork tapeworm	Niclosamide[†] or	Nausea, abdominal pain
		Praziquantel	Sedation, abdominal discomfort, fever, sweating, nausea, eosinophilia, photosensitivity, urticaria, abdominal pain, vomiting, and diarrhea
	Cysticercosis	Praziquantel (experimental) or surgery	Sedation, abdominal discomfort, fever, sweating, nausea, eosinophilia, photosensitivity, urticaria, abdominal pain, vomiting, and diarrhea
Toxocara canis	Visceral larval migrans	Thiabendazole or	**Nausea, vomiting, vertigo, rash,** leukopenial color vision disturbance, tinnitus, shock
		Diethylcarbamazine or	**GI disturbance**
		Mebendazole[†]	**GI disturbance**
Toxoplasma gondii	Toxoplasmosis (moderate to severe illness)	Pyrimethamine plus	**Folic acid deficiency,** blood dyscrasia, rash, vomiting, convulsions, shock; administer corticosteroids in ocular toxoplasmosis
		Sulfadiazine (teratogenic in animals) or	**Rash,** photosensitivity, hepatic and renal toxicity, blood dyscrasia, vasculitis
		Spiramycin	GI disturbance

Table continued on following page

Table 8–1. CHEMOTHERAPY OF PARASITIC DISEASES (Continued)

Infecting Organism	Disease	Chemotherapeutic Agent	Adverse Reactions*
	(immunosuppressed host)	Pyrimethamine plus	**Folic acid deficiency**, blood dyscrasia, rash, vomiting, convulsions, shock; administer corticosteroids in ocular toxoplasmosis
		Sulfadiazine plus Folinic acid	Rash, photosensitivity, hepatic and renal toxicity, blood dyscrasia, vasculitis
Trichinella spiralis	Trichinosis	Metronidazole[†]	**Nausea**, **headache**, **vomiting**, diarrhea, vertigo, insomnia, ataxia
Trichomonas vaginalis	Trichomoniasis	Metronidazole[†] or benzimidazole	**Nausea**, **headache**, **vomiting**, diarrhea, vertigo, insomnia, ataxia
Trichuris trichiura	Whipworm	Mebendazole[†]	**GI disturbance**
Trypanosoma cruzi	Chagas' disease	Nifurtimox[†,‡]	Nausea, dizziness, insomnia, peripheral neuropathy
Trypanosoma gambiense	West African sleeping sickness	Suramin[†,‡] or	**Rash**, **pruritus**, **vomiting**, **paresthesias**, shock, peripheral neuropathy
	Hemolymphatic disease	Pentamidine isethionate	**Breathlessness**, **dizziness**, **headache**, tachycardia, vomiting, itching
	CNS disease	Melarsoprol	**Encephalopathy**, vomiting, neuropathy, rash, myocarditis, hypertension
Trypanosoma brucei rhodesiense	East African sleeping sickness	Suramin[†,‡] or	**Rash**, **pruritus**, **vomiting**, paresthesias, shock, peripheral neuropathy
	Hemolymphatic disease	Pentamidine isethionate	**Breathlessness**, **dizziness**, **headache**, tachycardia, vomiting, itching
	CNS disease	Melarsoprol or	**Encephalopathy**, vomiting, neuropathy, rash, myocarditis, hypertension
		Tryparsamide and	**Nausea**, **vomiting**
		Suramin[†,‡]	**Rash**, **pruritus**, **vomiting**, **paresthesias**, shock, peripheral neuropathy
Wuchereria bancrofti	Filariasis; Bancroft's filariasis	Diethylcarbamazine or ivermectin[†]	**Allergic and febrile reactions** due to worm

*Most frequent adverse reactions to chemotherapy are noted in **boldface**.
[†]Not recommended for pregnant women or young children.
[‡]Available from CDC Drug Service, Centers for Disease Control and Prevention, Atlanta, GA 30333.

BIBLIOGRAPHY Altman, RM, et al: Control of *Culicoides* sand flies, Fort Kobbe Canal Zone in 1968. Mosquito News 30(2):235–240, 1970.

Anderson, RM, and May, RM: Helminthic infections of humans: Mathematical models, population dynamics, and control. Adv Parasitol 24:1–101, 1985.

Brabin, L, and Brabin, BJ: Parasitic infections in women and their consequences. Adv Parasitol 31:1–81, 1992.

Centers for Disease Control: Update: Chloroquine-resistant *Plasmodium falciparum*-Africa. MMWR 32(33):437–438, 1983.

Centers for Disease Control: Revised recommendations for preventing malaria in travelers to areas with chloroquine-resistant *Plasmodium falciparum*. Morbidity Mortality Weekly Report 14(4):185–190, 1985.

Crompton, DWT: Hookworm disease: Current status and new directions. Parasitology Today 5:1–2, 1989.

Cox, FEG (ed): *Modern Parasitology, ed 2. A Textbook of Parasitology,* ed2. Blackwell Scientific Publications, St Louis, 1993.

Davies, JB: Sixty years of onchocerciasis vector control: A chronologic summary with comments on eradication, reinvasion and insecticide resistance. Annu Rev Entomol 39:23–45, 1994.

Dye, C: Leishmaniasis epidemiology: The theory catches up. Parasitology 104(Suppl):S7–18, 1992.

Dye, C: The analysis of parasite transmission by bloodsucking insects. Annu Rev Entomol 37:1–19, 1992.

Goodwin, LG (ed): *Chemotherapy of Tropical Diseases: The Problem and the Challenge.* Wiley, Somerset, NJ, 1987.

Gustafsson, LL, and Abdi, YA (eds): *Handbook of Drugs for Tropical Parasitic Infections.* Taylor & Francis, Bristol, PA, 1987.

Kierszenbaum, F (ed): *Parasitic Infections and the Immune System.* Academic Press, San Diego, 1994.

Lane, RP: The contribution of sandfly control to leishmaniasis control. Ann Soc Belg Med Trop 71(suppl)1:65–74, 1991.

Liew, FY (ed): *Vaccination Strategies of Tropical Diseases.* CRC Press, Boca Raton, FL, 1989.

The Medical Letter, Inc: Drugs for parasitic infections. January 31, 1986, pp 9–17.

The Medical Letter, Inc: Drugs for parasitic infections. February 12, 1988, pp 15–24.

Miller, MJ, and Love, EJ (eds): *Parasitic Diseases: Treatment and Control.* CRC Press, Boca Raton, FL, 1989.

Pampano, E: *A Textbook of Malaria Eradication.* Oxford University Press, London, 1963.

Pearson, R, and Guerrant, R: Praziquantel: A major advance in antihelminthic therapy. Ann Intern Med 99:195, 1983.

Physicians Desk Reference, ed 48. Medical Economics, Orasill, NJ, 1994.

Proceedings of a Symposium of the International Atomic Energy Commission: Sterile insect technique and radiation in insect control. June 29–July 3, 1981, United Nations, New York, 1982.

Schultz, MG: Current Concepts in Parasitology: Parasitic Diseases. N Engl J Med 297:1259–1261, 1977.

Soulsby, EJL: *Immune Responses in Parasitic Infections: Immunology, Immunopathology and Immunoprophylaxis* (4 Vols). CRC Press, Boca Raton, FL, 1986.

Warren, KS: *Immunology and Molecular Biology of Parasitic Infections,* ed 3. Blackwell Scientific Publications, Oxford, 1992.

Wyngaarden, LB, and Smith, LH: *Cecil Textbook of Medicine,* ed 19. WB Saunders, Philadelphia, 1992.

Final Examination

Using separate sheets of paper, answer the following questions. Allow 90 minutes to complete this text. **Except when indicated, all questions are worth 1 point each.** A satisfactory score is 80 percent or more. Answers are given in the next section.

1. State the scientific name for the parasites illustrated below. **(5 points)**

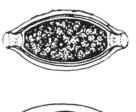

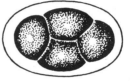

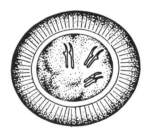

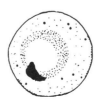

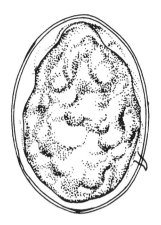

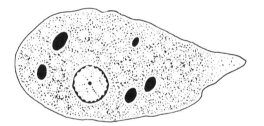

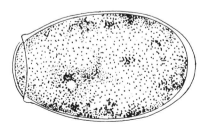

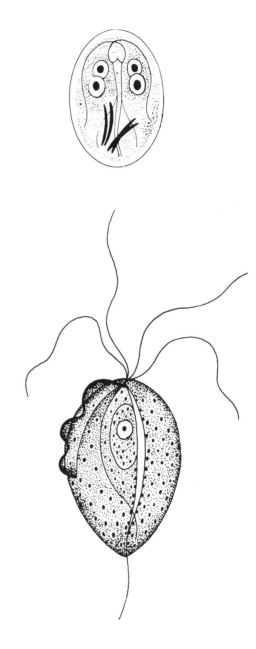

2. Draw the life cycle for each parasite given below. **(10 points)**
   a. *Ascaris lumbricoides*
   b. *Diphyllobothrium latum*
   c. *Trypanosoma cruzi*
   d. *Enterobius vermicularis*
   e. *Leishmania donovani*

3. A patient was treated with immunosuppressants during a kidney transplant and subsequently exhibited symptoms of two parasitic infections. Which were they? **(2 points)**
   a. *Ascaris lumbricoides*
   b. *Toxoplasma gondii*
   c. *Schistosoma mansoni*
   d. *Strongyloides stercoralis*
   e. *Plasmodium falciparum*

4. Which one of the following parasites is *not* found most prevalently in North or South America?
   a. *Trypanosoma cruzi*
   b. *Leishmania braziliensis*
   c. *Necator americanus*
   d. *Mansonella ozzardi*
   e. *Paragonimus westermani*

5. For each parasite given, select its most common body location in humans. Choices may be used more than once. **(5 points)**

   a. _____ *Schistosoma mansoni*
   b. _____ *Clonorchis sinensis*
   c. _____ *Trichura trichiura*
   d. _____ *Leishmania braziliensis*
   e. _____ *Trypanosoma b. rhodesiense*
   f. _____ *Echinococcus granulosus*
   g. _____ *Endolimax nana*
   h. _____ *Plasmodium vivax*
   i. _____ *Strongyloides stercoralis*
   j. _____ *Loa loa*

   1. blood
   2. liver
   3. intestine
   4. striated muscle
   5. skin
   6. lymph nodes
   7. heart muscle
   8. eye
   9. bladder veins
   10. intestinal veins
   11. subcutaneous tissue
   12. macrophages

6. The intermediate host for *Taenia saginata* is:
   a. Pig
   b. Cow
   c. Human
   d. Bear
   e. Sheep

7. Which of the following are the diagnostic morphologic characteristics for *Entamoeba histolytica*? (Choose all that apply.)
   a. Centrally located karyosome
   b. A micronucleus and macronucleus
   c. Large glycogen vacuole
   d. Flagella
   e. Large karyosome with a faintly visible nuclear membrane
   f. Ingested red blood cells

8. Which of the following require no intermediate host? (Choose all that apply.)
   a. *Hymenolepis nana*
   b. *Giardia lamblia*
   c. *Strongyloides stercoralis*
   d. *Trichuris trichiura*
   e. *Schistosoma mansoni*

9. Which cestode produces an operculated egg?
   a. *Taenia saginata*
   b. *Hymenolepis nana*
   c. *Diphyllobothrium latum*
   d. *Echinococcus granulosus*
   e. *Taenia solium*

10. A stained blood smear reveals giant platelets and many reticulocytes containing Schüffner's dots, large ring forms, and schizonts with 12 to 24 merozoites. You would name this as:

a. *Plasmodium vivax*
b. *Plasmodium falciparum*
c. *Plasmodium ovale*
d. *Plasmodium malariae*
e. *Babesia* spp.

11. When purged specimens are to be examined for amebae, which of the following should be used to obtain the specimen?
    a. Barium salts
    b. Castor oil
    c. Fleet Phospho-Soda
    d. Mineral oil

12. A stained fecal smear reveals mononucleate flagellates with a comma-shaped posterior, and lemon-shaped mononucleate cysts with a clear, nipplelike bleb at one end. You would name this as:
    a. *Trichomonas hominis*
    b. *Chilomastix mesnili*
    c. *Trichomonas vaginalis*
    d. *Giardia lamblia*
    e. *Endolimax nana*

13. Infection with *Brugia malayi* is best diagnosed by:
    a. Zinc-sulfate flotation concentration
    b. Cellophane tape test
    c. Xenodiagnosis
    d. Trichrome staining of a fecal smear
    e. Knott concentration test

14. All but one of the following are methods of human infection with *Toxoplasma gondii*. Which of the following is *not* a method of toxoplasmosis infection?
    a. Mosquito bite
    b. In utero transmission
    c. Ingestion of oocyst
    d. Ingestion of pseudocyst in meat
    e. Ingestion of trachyzoite in milk

15. Which of the following conditions is *not* a zoonotic infection?
    a. Scabies
    b. Swimmer's itch
    c. Tropical eosinophilic lung
    d. Visceral larval migrans
    e. Cutaneous larval migrans

16. Patient traveled last summer to Africa and has a spiking fever every third day. A stained blood smear reveals:

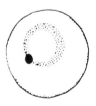

The parasite causing this infection is:
    a. *Plasmodium vivax*
    b. *Plasmodium malariae*
    c. *Plasmodium falciparum*
    d. *Plasmodium ovale*

17. Cercariae of this parasite penetrate the skin of humans, thereby causing infection.
    a. *Fasciolopsis buski*
    b. *Heterophyes heterophyes*
    c. *Schistosoma japonicum*
    d. *Paragonimus westermani*

18. These two infections were found by stool examination of a child who had a history of eating dirt. (2 points)
    a. *Trichinella spiralis*
    b. *Ascaris lumbricoides*
    c. *Paragonimus westermani*
    d. *Trichuris trichiura*
    e. *Taenia solium*

19. Recovery in human feces of a 7-mm-long gravid proglottid containing 8 lateral uterine branches indicates infection with:
    a. *Hymenolepis nana*
    b. *Diphyllobothrium latum*
    c. *Echinococcus granulosus*
    d. *Taenia saginata*
    e. *Taenia solium*

20. This parasite was found in the blood smear of a patient who had a recent summer vacation in New England and reported many insect and tick bites.
    a. *Plasmodium vivax*
    b. AIDS virus
    c. *Phthirus pubis*
    d. *Babesia* spp.

21. Pinworm disease can be best diagnosed by using:
    a. The formalin-ethyl acetate concentration method
    b. The cellophane tape test
    c. A direct fecal smear preparation
    d. None of the above

22. A small, operculated egg with a light bulb shape was found in the feces of a patient with liver abnormalities.
    a. *Fasciola hepatica*
    b. *Paragonimus westermani*
    c. *Fasciolopsis buski*
    d. *Clonorchis sinensis*

23. Mature trophozoites and young schizonts in blood smear show a distinct tendency toward band formation and the red blood cells are not enlarged.
    a. *Plasmodium vivax*
    b. *Plasmodium malariae*
    c. *Plasmodium falciparum*
    d. *Plasmodium ovale*

24. Found in the feces of a patient complaining of abdominal distress and diarrhea.
    a. *Giardia lamblia*
    b. *Trichomonas vaginalis*
    c. *Chilomastix mesnili*
    d. *Trichomonas tenax*

25. Only one of the following parasites produces eggs that are immediately infective to humans, and the eggs infect a person directly via ingestion. Which is it?
    a. *Schistosoma mansoni*
    b. *Enterobius vermicularis*
    c. *Trichuris trichiura*
    d. *Clonorchis sinensis*
    e. *Taenia saginata*

26. Match the arthropod vectors with the appropriate organism. **(5 points)**

    a. _____ mosquito (*Culex* spp.)

    b. _____ black fly (*Simulium* spp.)

    c. _____ mango fly (*Chrysops* spp.)

    d. _____ crustacean (*Cyclops* spp.)

    e. _____ tsetse fly (*Glossina* spp.)

    1. *Loa loa*
    2. *Onchocerca volvulus*
    3. *Trypanosoma b. rhodesiense*
    4. *Diphyllobothrium latum*
    5. *Wuchereria bancrofti*

27. Which of the following intestinal protozoa is *not* identified as a causative agent of diarrhea?
    a. *Entamoeba histolytica*
    b. *Dientamoeba fragilis*
    c. *Giardia lamblia*
    d. *Balantidium coli*
    e. *Entamoeba coli*

28. Identified from the bloody sputum of an immigrant from the Far East:
    a. *Fasciola hepatica*
    b. *Clonorchis sinensis*
    c. *Paragonimus westermani*
    d. *Fasciolopsis buski*

29. Control of a flea infestation is different from control of lice. Why?
    a. Fleas are much more resistant to insecticides.
    b. Fleas reproduce off the host, laying eggs in the environment.
    c. Fleas are larger than lice.
    d. Fleas don't need a blood meal.

30. In clinical cases of *Wuchereria bancrofti,* the most favorable time to find parasites in the blood is:
    a. Early morning
    b. Middle of the night
    c. During late afternoon
    d. Any time

31. Match the disease with the causative parasite. **(4 points)**

    a. _____ creeping eruption

    b. _____ visceral larval migrans

    c. _____ tropical eosinophilia

    d. _____ eosinophilic meningitis

    1. *Dirofilaria* spp.
    2. *Anisakis* spp.
    3. *Angiostrongylus* spp.
    4. *Toxocara* spp.
    5. *Ancylostoma caninum*

32. All of the following except one are best diagnosed by identification in a blood smear. Which one is not?
    a. *Trypanosoma b. gambiense*
    b. *Babesia microti*
    c. *Plasmodium falciparum*
    d. *Onchocerca volvulus*
    e. *Wuchereria bancrofti*

33. All of the following, except one, infect humans by entrance of the infective stage through the skin. Which one has a different route of entrance?
    a. *Schistosoma japonicum*
    b. *Strongyloides stercoralis*
    c. *Ancylostoma duodenale*
    d. *Necator americanus*
    e. *Heterophyes heterophyes*

34. Match the following with the appropriate question. **(10 points)**
    1. *Entamoeba histolytica*
    2. *Entamoeba coli*
    3. *Endolimax nana*
    4. *Iodamoeba bütschlii*
    5. *Dientamoeba fragilis*

    a. _____ Which ameba trophozoite feeds on red blood cells?

    b. _____ Which ameba has a nucleus with a heavy chromatin ring and an eccentrically located karyosome?

    c. _____ Which ameba has a nucleus with an even chromatin ring and a centrally located karyosome?

    d. _____ Which ameba has up to four nuclei in a round cyst?

    e. _____ Which ameba cyst contains a glycogen vacuole?

    f. _____ Which ameba has a nucleus with a large karyosome and a chromatin ring that is not visible?

    g. _____ Which ameba does not form cysts?

    h. _____ Which ameba causes intestinal ulcers and bloody dysentery?

    i. _____ Which ameba can invade the liver and cause pathology in that organ?

    j. _____ Which ameba forms the smallest cyst?

35. The trichrome stain is used to identify:
    a. Blood protozoa
    b. Helminth eggs in feces
    c. Intestinal protozoa
    d. Antibodies to tissue parasites

36. Below are listed sources of error that may have impact on a quality smear stained for parasites. Identify which one is *not* a source of error.
    a. Blood smear too thick
    b. Blood smear too new
    c. Stain buffer has wrong pH
    d. Wrong timing during staining

37. The head of the scolex of *Diphyllobothrium latum*:
    a. Is armed with hooks
    b. Has a retractable rostellum
    c. Has four suckers
    d. Has two sucking grooves

38. Egg has a large lateral spine.
    a. *Schistosoma haematobium*
    b. *Clonorchis sinensis*
    c. *Fasciola hepatica*
    d. *Schistosoma mansoni*

39. Which of the following is the best transport preservative for protozoa or flagellate trophozoites?
    a. Zinc sulfate
    b. Formalin and ethyl acetate
    c. Polyvinyl alcohol
    d. Iodine

40. The cysticercus larva form is found where noted as part of the life cycle of which parasite?
    a. On aquatic vegetation; *Fasciola hepatica*
    b. In fish muscle; *Diphyllobothrium latum*
    c. In pork muscle; *Taenia solium*
    d. In mosquitoes; *Dracunculus medinensis*

41. Which of these Platyhelminthes infect humans through ingestion of undercooked fish? (You may choose more than one answer.) **(5 points)**
    a. *Clonorchis sinensis*
    b. *Paragonimus westermani*
    c. *Diphyllobothrium latum*
    d. *Heterophyes heterophyes*
    e. *Schistosoma mansoni*
    f. *Echinococcus granulosus*

42. *Babesia* spp. is transmitted to humans:
    a. By the bite of an infected tick
    b. By the bite of an infected fly (*Chrysops* spp.)
    c. By ingestion of a cyst
    d. By the bite of an infected mosquito (*Anopheles* spp.)

43. Name two zoonotic infections caused by: **(6 points)**
    a. Nematodes
    b. Protozoa
    c. Platyhelminthes

44. Which of the following causes primary amebic meningoencephalitis?
    a. *Entamoeba histolytica*
    b. *Babesia* spp.
    c. *Naegleria* spp.
    d. *Sarcocystis* spp.
    e. *Acanthamoeba* spp.

45. Because you are responsible for parasite control on an island, you chemically treat the small freshwater lake for snails, but you accidently dump in too much chemical and kill every living thing in the lake. Your action breaks the life cycle and controls the spread of which of the following parasites? (Choose all correct answers.) **(5 points)**
    a. *Fasciolopis buski*
    b. *Taenia solium*
    c. *Schistosoma mansoni*
    d. *Diphyllobothrium latum*
    e. *Hymenolepis nana*

46. Which of the following requires two different intermediate hosts in its life cycle?
    a. *Clonorchis sinensis*
    b. *Schistosoma mansoni*
    c. *Trichuris trichiura*
    d. *Loa loa*
    e. *Echinococcus granulosus*

47. Which of the following exhibits diurnal periodicity?
    a. *Wuchereria bancrofti*
    b. *Brugia malayi*
    c. *Loa loa*
    d. *Onchocerca volvulus*

48. Below is shown the final centrifuge tube appearance for two different concentration techniques. Indicate where the parasites are found in each tube and state what concentration technique each tube represents. **(5 points)**

A.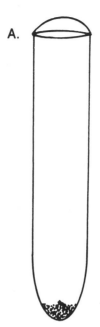

B.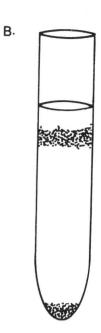

Answer Key

CHAPTER 1 (PRE-TEST)

1. b
2. d
3. c
4. c
5. c

6. a
7. d
8. b
9. a
10. c

11. a = 3; b = 5; c = 1; d = 2; e = 4

12. a. **Vector:** any arthropod or other living carrier that transports a pathogenic micro-organism from an infected to a noninfected host.
    b. **Host:** the species of animal or plant that harbors a parasite and provides some metabolic resources to the parasitic species.
    c. **Proglottid:** one of the segments of a tapeworm; each contains male and female reproductive organs when mature.
    d. **Definitive host:** animal in which a parasite passes its adult existence and/or sexual reproduction phase.
    e. **Operculum:** the lid or caplike cover on certain helminth eggs.

CHAPTER 2   1.

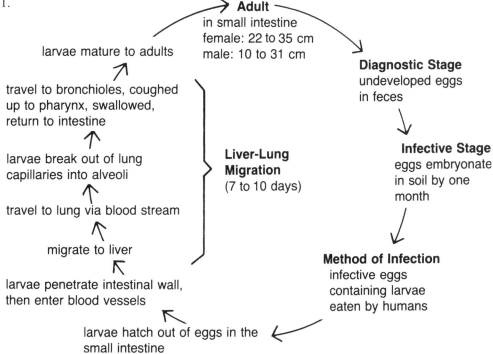

2. a. *Wuchereria bancrofti*
   b. *Culex* or *Anopheles* spp. mosquito
   c. Blood specimen, stained thick and thin smears. Concentrate the specimen by centrifugation. Serology helpful also.

3. a. **Cutaneous larval migrans.** A disease caused by the migration of larvae of *Ancylostoma* spp. (dog or cat hookworm) or other helminths under the skin of humans. Larval migration is marked by thin, red papular lines of eruption. Also termed creeping eruption.
   b. **Diurnal.** Occurring during the daytime.
   c. **Diagnostic stage.** A developmental stage of the pathogenic organism that can be detected in human body secretions, discharges, feces, blood, or tissue by chemical means or microscopic observation as an aid in diagnosis.
   d. **Infective stage.** The stage of a parasite at which it is capable of entering the host and continuing development within the host.
   e. **Prepatent stage.** The time elapsing between initial infection with the parasite and reproduction by the mature parasite.

4. d	7. d
5. b	8. b
6. a	9. c

CHAPTER 3   1. a. **Hexacanth embryo.** A tapeworm larva having six hooklets; also termed **onchosphere**; found in all *Taenia* spp. eggs.
   b. **Hermaphroditic.** Having both male and female reproductive organs within the same individual. All tapeworms have both sets of reproductive organs in each segment of the adult (i.e., all adult tapeworms are hermaphroditic).
   c. **"Armed" scolex.** Crown of hooks on anterior end of a tapeworm; causes attachment to the wall of the intestine of a host by means of suckers and hooks (e.g., *Taenia solium*).
   d. **Proglottid.** One of the segments of a tapeworm (all adult tapeworms form proglottids). Each proglottid contains male and female reproductive organs when mature.
   e. **Hydatid cyst.** A vesicular structure formed by *Echinococcus granulosus* larvae in the intermediate host; contains fluid, brood capsules, and also daughter cysts in which the scolices of potential tapeworms are formed.

2. a. 5 (4)   d. 2, 1
   b. 4   e. 10 (4)
   c. 7

3.   a. *Hymenolepis nana*

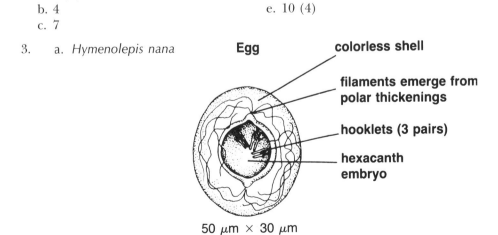

Egg

colorless shell

filaments emerge from polar thickenings

hooklets (3 pairs)

hexacanth embryo

50 μm × 30 μm

b. *Diphyllobothrium latum*

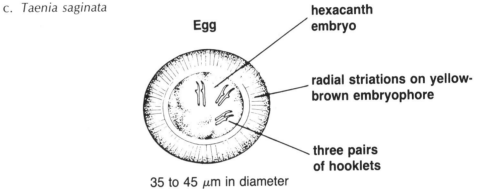

Egg

terminal (abopercular) knob

coracidium (undeveloped embryo)

operculum

75 μm × 45 μm

c. *Taenia saginata*

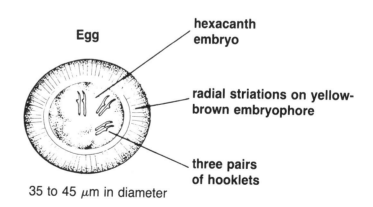

Egg

hexacanth embryo

radial striations on yellow-brown embryophore

three pairs of hooklets

35 to 45 μm in diameter

d. *Taenia solium*

Egg

hexacanth embryo

radial striations on yellow-brown embryophore

three pairs of hooklets

35 to 45 μm in diameter

e. *Echinococcus granulosus*

Hydatid cyst (partial cross-section)

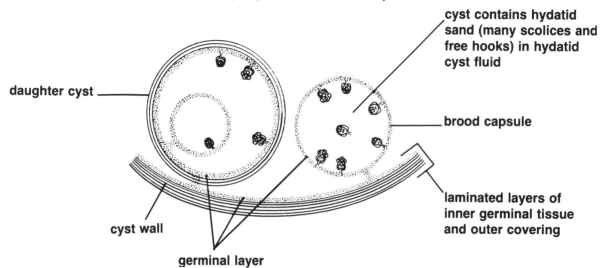

daughter cyst

cyst contains hydatid sand (many scolices and free hooks) in hydatid cyst fluid

brood capsule

laminated layers of inner germinal tissue and outer covering

cyst wall

germinal layer

4. a. 6	e. 8
b. 2	f. 7
c. 5	g. 3
d. 1	h. 4
5. a	7. c
6. c	8. b

CHAPTER 4

1. 1 egg   6 metacercaria   2 miracidium   4 redia
   7 adult   3 sporocyst   5 cercaria

2. D. Possible contact with sheep-transmitted, sheepdog-transmitted, and freshwater fish-transmitted parasites.
   a. No contact with pigs. No contact with snails or fish hosts of Oriental lung fluke.
   b. No contact with snails that host *S. mansoni* or hosts of *C. sinensis*.
   c. No contact with snail hosts of *S. japonicum*.
   d. No contact with snails or fish hosts of *H. heterophyes*.

3. a. 1. *Fasciolopsis buski* (large intestinal fluke) ingestion
      2. *Clonorchis sinensis* (Chinese liver fluke)
      3. *Schistosoma mansoni* (Manson's blood fluke)
   b. 1. Human eats metacercariae on uncooked water plant
      2. Human eats metacercariae on uncooked fish
      3. Cercariae penetrate skin

4. Method of infection with blood flukes (schistosomes) is by penetration of the skin by cercariae in fresh water. Prevention of infection with blood flukes therefore requires prohibiting human feces or urine from contaminating fresh water, snail control, not entering contaminated water without protection, treating carriers with drugs, and education.

   Prevention of infection with intestinal flukes requires cooking all fish and crustaceans thoroughly, washing water plants such as watercress and water chestnuts thoroughly, education about methods of infection as well as education about not contaminating fresh water with human waste, treating carriers, and snail control.

5. d

7. b

6. c

CHAPTER 5
1. a. 4
   b. 7
   c. 14
   d. 8
   e. 11
   f. 5, 1, 2

   g. 2
   h. 9, 10
   i. 1
   j. 3
   k. 6
   l. 12

2. In trophozoite: Study differential characteristics of size, consistency and inclusions (bacterial or red blood cells) in cytoplasm, directional vs. random motility, shape of pseudopodia, staining characteristics of nuclear structures. In cysts: study differential characteristics of size, number of nuclei and nuclear structure, shape of chromatoid bodies, vacuoles.

3. a. **Trophozoite.** The motile stage of a protozoon that feeds, multiplies, and maintains the colony within the host.
   b. **Cyst.** The immotile stage protected by a cyst wall formed by the parasite. In this stage, the protozoon is readily transmitted to a new host.
   c. **Sporozoite.** The form of *Plasmodium* that develops inside the sporocyst, invades the salivary glands of the mosquito, and is transmitted to humans.
   d. **Schizogony.** Asexual multiplication of *Apicomplexa*; multiple intracellular nuclear division precedes cytoplasmic division.
   e. **Carrier.** A host harboring and disseminating a parasite but exhibiting no clinical signs or symptoms.
   f. **Oocyst.** The encysted form of the ookinete; occurs on the stomach wall of *Anopheles* spp. mosquitoes infected with malaria.
   g. **Pseudocyst.** A cystlike structure formed by the host during an acute infection with *Toxoplasma gondii*. The cyst is filled with tachyzoites in normal hosts; may occur in brain or other tissues. Latent source of infection that may become active if immunosuppression occurs.
   h. **L.D. body (Leishman-Donovan body).** Each of the small ovoid amastigote forms found in tissue macrophages of the liver and spleen in patients with *Leishmania donovani* infection.
   i. **Paroxysm.** The fever-chills syndrome in malaria. Spiking fever corresponds to the release of merozoites and toxic materials from the parasitized red blood cell (RBC), and shaking chills occur during schizont development. Occurs in malaria cyclically every 36 to 72 hours, depending on the species.
   j. **Atrium** (pl. **atria**). An opening; in a human, refers to the mouth, vagina, and urethra.

4. a. Bite of *Phlebotomus* spp.
   b. Ingestion of cyst in contaminated water or food
   c. Infected feces of *Triatoma* spp. rubbed into bite or conjunctiva
   d. Ingestion of oocyst, trophozoite, or pseudocyst; congenital transmission
   e. In men, sexual intercourse; in women, contamination with infectious material from vagina
   f. Ingestion of cyst in contaminated water or food
   g. Tick bite
   h. Bite of *Anopheles* mosquito; contaminated blood injection
   i. Bite of *Glossina* spp.
   j. Bite of *Phlebotomus* spp.

5. *P. vivax*

**Trophozoite
(single ring)**

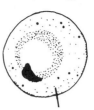

Schüffner's dots

**Note: Single ring,
one-third diameter of
an RBC; invades only
immature RBCs so that
large bluish cells are
parasitized.
RBC shows red-stained
Schüffner's dots which
become visible between
15 and 20 hours following
invasion of the cell.**

P. malariae

**Trophozoite
(single ring)**

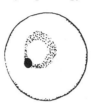

**Note: Trophozoite
forms band across RBC
during early schizogony.**

Trophozoites

P. falciparum

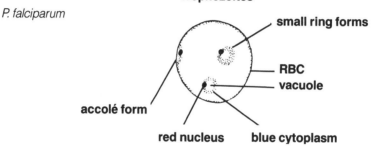

small ring forms

RBC

vacuole

accolé form

red nucleus   **blue cytoplasm**

6. a	9. d
7. d	10. e
8. b	11. e

CHAPTER 6

1. a. 5
   b. 6
   c. 1
   d. 3
   e. 2

2. a. 5
   b. 1, 2, 3, 4, 5, 7
   c. 4
   d. 6
   e. 5
   f. 3
   g. 3
   h. 1
   i. 7
   j. 3

3. All flea stages develop to maturity in the environment rather than on the host, as is the case with lice. Therefore, treatment for fleas must include chemically treating the rooms of the house as well as the host. For lice, primary treatment is to the infected

individual, although personal items such as combs, bedding, and towels must also be disinfected.

4. Annoyance, allergic reaction, blood loss, toxins or venom in bites, secondary bacterial infections, transmission of a variety of microorganisms by mechanical or biologic methods, loss of food crops, loss of animal productivity, myiasis.

5. d   8. e

6. b   9. c

7. a

CHAPTER 7   1. False—1 or 2 is sufficient for helminths, 3 to 6 for suspected amebiasis or giardiasis.

2. True

3. False—not all intestinal protozoa form cysts; trophozoites die and hookworm eggs may hatch if specimen is not rapidly preserved.

4. True

5. False—oil enemas make examination impossible.

6. False—other species of parasites may also be present.

7. False—parasitemia may be too low. Thick smears are recommended in addition to thin smears.

8. Low light for contrast; unstained amebae are translucent.

9. First thing in the morning before washing or defecation because generally pinworms deposit eggs at night.

10. Formalin-ethyl acetate; sedimentation of parasite stages. Zinc sulfate; flotation, based on differential specific gravity of parasite and the liquid medium. For procedures, see pages 126–130.

11. 1.18 to 1.20; hydrometer

12. Schistosome eggs, infertile ascaris eggs, operculated eggs

13. Ether or ethyl acetate

14. Thin: little distortion, but hard to find the parasites. Thick: distortion, but easier to find parasites.

15. Place slide in distilled water until hemoglobin color disappears from slide.

16. Cytoplasm light blue-green or pink for *E. histolytica*, more purple for *E. coli*. Karyosomes stain ruby red.

17. Boeck-Drbohlav, Balamuth, Cleveland-Collier. Add sterile rice powder and stool to media. Incubate at 37°C for 24 hours; examine top of sediment for trophozoites.

18. Disodium phosphate and monosodium phosphate, ph 7.0

19. a. 2, 4   f. 4
    b. 1, 5   g. 8
    c. 6   h. 7
    d. 4   i. 4
    e. 3   j. 7

20. d   23. c

21. d   24. b

22. a   25. b

FINAL EXAMINATION

1. *Trichuris trichiura*
   Necator americanus (or *Ancylostoma braziliense*)
   Taenia solium or *Taenia saginata*
   Ascaris lumbricoides
   Plasmodium vivax
   Schistosoma japonicum
   Entamoeba histolytica
   Paragonimus westermani
   Giardia lamblia
   Trichomonis vaginalis

2. a—Diagram 2–4 (page 15); c—Diagram 5–6 (page 81); e—Diagram 5–7 (page 83); b—Diagram 3–3 (page 40); d—Diagram 2–2 (page 12)

3. b, d

4. e

5. a = 10; b = 2; c = 3; d = 12, 5, 11; e = 1; f = 2; g = 3; h = 1,(2); i = 3; j = 8, 1

6. b

7. a, f

8. a, b, c, d

9. c

10. a

11. c

12. b

13. e

14. a

15. a

16. b

17. c

18. b, d

19. e

20. d

21. b

22. d

23. b

24. a

25. b

26. a = 5; b = 2; c = 1; d = 4; e = 3

27. e

28. c

29. b

30. b

31. a = 5; b = 4; c = 1; d = 3

32. d

33. e

34. a = 1; b = 2; c = 1; d = 1; e = 4; f = 3; g = 5; h = 1; i = 1; j = 3

35. c

36. b

37. d

38. d

39. c

40. c

41. a, c, d

42. a

43. a. *Ancylostoma* spp., *Angiostrongylus* spp., *Anisakis* spp., *Capillaria philippinensis*, *Dirofilaria* spp., *Gnathostoma* spp., *Gongylonema pulchrum*, *Thelazia* spp., *Toxocara* spp.
    b. *Trypanosoma* spp., *Sarcocystis* spp., *Leishmania* spp., *Toxoplasma gondii*, *Babesia* spp.
    c. *Fasciola hepatica*, swimmer's itch, *Echinococcus granulosus*, *Hymenolepis diminuta*, *Dipylidium caninum*, sparganosis, cysticercosis

44. e

45. a, c, d

46. a

47. c

48. a. Parasites at the top of the fluid: flotation method
    b. Parasites at the bottom of the tube: sedimentation method

Index

An "f" following a page number indicates a diagram or an illustration. A "t" following a page number indicates a table. A number in **boldface** indicates a color plate.